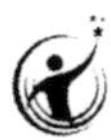

A Wealth of Health

Join the health movement & thrive

By Ursula Kaiser & Patricia Acerra

www.ursulakaiser.com

DISCLAIMER

The statements made about products and services have not been evaluated by the US Food and Drug Administration. They are not intended to diagnose, treat, cure, or prevent any condition or disease. Please consult with your own physician or health care specialist regarding the suggestions and recommendations made in this book. Except where specifically stated neither Author or Publisher nor any other contributors or other representatives will be liable for damages arising out of or in connection with the use of this book. This is a comprehensive limitation of liability that applies to all damages of any kind, including without limitation compensatory, direct, indirect, or consequential damages, loss of date, income or profit, loss of or damage to property and claims of third parties.You must understand that this book is not intended as a substitute for consultation with a licensed healthcare practitioner, such as your physician. Before you begin any healthcare program, or change your lifestyle in any way, you should consult your physician or other licensed healthcare practitioner to insure that you are in good health and that the examples contained in this book will not harm you. This book provides the reader content related to topics concerning physical and or mental health issues. As such, use of this book implies your acceptance of this disclaimer.

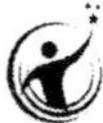

BIO AND INTRODUCTION

Health should not be a whirlwind of science studies and trends. Health should be simple and natural. By providing you with an easy education based on ancient wisdom and common sense, we hope to enable you to quickly cut through all the hype and the trends that you are being bombarded with every day. By the end of this book, you will be able to make informed decisions on the spot that will support your goal to live a vibrant and healthy life.

Don't be too hard on yourself. Apply the 80/20 rule and know that if you're following 80% of what we suggest here, you'll be way ahead of the curve.

Look, we know that by urging you to view the way you eat differently we are asking you to change half of your lifestyle. The other half of your lifestyle is how you think, and you are in control of changing that, too. We are encouraging you to be more responsible for your health, and if you have this book in your hands, then obviously you are somewhat open-minded to it. Try something different for 30 days. Just 30 days, and you will see a positive change in your habits. We believe in you, but more importantly YOU need to believe in YOU!

We want you to succeed. For every one person who succeeds at a healthier lifestyle, at least two or three of their friends will follow suit. When people see how vibrant and energetic you have become they are going to want to get on the bandwagon, too. We can begin a world health movement.

It doesn't matter what diseases run in your family or what shape you're in right now; the same principles of health apply. You begin a journey with one step. Then you take another and another. With small steps of common sense education, you will easily be able to understand why to choose one food or one behavior over another on your road to optimal health.

The bookshelves are stacked high with hundreds, if not thousands, of diets and theories on health and longevity. It's confusing. It's overwhelming. We want you to simply concentrate on the basics and see how they resonate with you. If you just start by learning some very simple principles, you will be able to weed out new fads like an expert gardener.

Written by Ursula Kaiser and Patricia Acerra. URSULA KAISER is an author and national public speaker on the topics of health and healing. A small-town girl from Germany, she dreamed big, came to the United States and started her own global kitchen utensil business. She appeared on shows such as *Good Morning America*, and designed and sold baking products to Martha Stewart.

In 1999, she was diagnosed with ovarian cancer, and doctors gave her three months to live. How could this be? Ursula had always prided herself on being strong, healthy and balanced; health food, tennis, skiing, biking and rollerblading were regular parts of her life. However, a long-standing lawsuit injected heavy stress into her mind and body. She was certain that the stress had attracted the cancer, pure and simple. Not interested in the devastating side effects of chemotherapy and radiation, Ursula chose to use holistic medicine to heal herself. She came away, and remains cancer free and has spent 15 years investigating and trying many alternative solutions to keep her health. She is now passionately committed to giving back and helping others overcome illness through holistic approaches. In this book, she shares some of what she learned on her journey to wellness.

PATRICIA ACERRA, Dipl.Ac. (NCCAOM), CCHt, is a nationally certified Acupuncture Physician and Certified Clinical and Transpersonal Hypnotherapist who has held a private practice in Naples, Florida for over 20 years.

Through the challenges brought to her by her patients, and constant research for solutions, it became clearer and clearer to her that the basics are what really matter. Physical, mental and emotional health is intertwined in the fabric of daily life. What you do on a daily basis has the largest impact on your health. Prevention is key. It makes no sense to incorporate healing remedies into your lifestyle without eliminating the things that are making you ill. She found that once her patients understood how their bodies were crying out for help, they were their own best doctors. You cannot feel like a victim. You must empower yourself.

Ursula and Patricia met over 15 years ago at a Hawaiian Huna Cleanse and have been friends ever since. They combine their knowledge and experience now to provide you with a practical guide to achieving and maintaining wonderful health in the midst of a world filled with conflicting information, busy schedules and toxins and stress around every corner.

The inspiration for this book title, ***A Wealth of Health***, Join the Health Movement and Thrive comes from noticing (and being amazed by) people we continuously meet in their 90's who are vibrant, thriving and happy. Patricia's mother, Anne, always said, "Just live, love and laugh if you want to get along." But, when asked to offer us their "secrets" of how they stayed so healthy and engaged well past the average human, their reasons varied.

For example, Emery took up rowing when he was 65. He is 93 now – still rowing – with quite a few medals under his belt. Patricia's Mom, Anne, who is 93 years old, still enjoys dancing as much as she has her entire life – and gets a kick out of being a fashionista (heels and all). We all know of someone past his or her 80s with a healthy heart and a zest for life and each reason is different. Yet, in summary, the order of important aspects of staying healthy repeatedly showed the following:

1. Be Happy and have a social network.
2. Have a passion – even if it is only your hobby.
3. Exercise – stay active.
4. Eat good food!

"What is called genius is the abundance of life and health."

— Henry David Thoreau

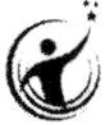

FORWARD

Dr. Pat Sager Lane, Jacksonville, FL

This very valuable "how to be and stay healthy" guidebook could not be written at a more appropriate time. We are in an epidemic of dis-ease and unwillingness worldwide. According to the World Health Organization, WHO, we are in a global health crisis (World Health Organization & Food and Agriculture Organization of the United States, 2003, Diet, Nutrition and the Prevention of Chronic Diseases).

The obvious signs of this global health crisis are revealed in major increases in the numbers of people of all ages suffering from chronic diseases like autism, obesity, metabolic syndrome, multiple sclerosis, Parkinson's disease, and diabetes. Many types of dementia, of which Alzheimer's is the most recognizable, may be included in this neurological melee. As a gerontologist, who was born in and lives in Florida, I felt it appropriate to study the process of aging in this state. Florida is often referred to as "God's waiting room". It made sense to study the impact of aging on health in my home state.

I was also led to study nutritional choices and their impact on health and aging. I was having symptoms of pre-diabetes. My new husband was a diabetic with worsening symptoms, taking multiple high dosage prescription medications for diabetes as prescribed, and eating no sugars. I began to see the correlations in the devastating results of poor dietary and life style choices in seniors (those from 55-65 years old) and in older-older adults (65-95 years old).

Good nutrition must include correct food and nutrient choices. Prepackaged and Fast Food is not a food group. Correct food choices do matter as to the quality of life as we age. They become our wealth in how they affect our medical outcomes and financial resources at all ages. Medical care is expensive and can mean loss of income for an older or younger disabled adult or child, and for their family members, who may need to become full time caregivers. This book can ward off the devastating effects resulting from future disability and the associated extreme expenses. Preventative measures such as life style choices, recommended by this book, are the best insurance plan to protect your health as your wealth of tomorrow. Good health is your true asset protection. It will allow you a quality of life with mobility and clear thinking for fun experiences as a full participant, not just as a bystander, as you grow older. So how do you choose what is best to consume as the best food choices and best life style changes to enhance and expand your quality and length of life? Unfortunately, in my questioning of many people about what they choose to eat, I have discovered they make their choices based on hype, myth, and habit. My research and observations have led to my book on this subject to be released in 2015. Many people are duped into eating what the food advertisers tell them is best for them, or what looks appealing in commercials. The latest crazes of low fat, no fat, no eggs, no bacon with nitrates, no salt, and no sugar promote buying products that use artificial sweeteners to cut calories, etc. Many of the artificial sweeteners are themselves harmful to our health since they are derived from chemicals. Earning my doctorate degree taught me more than the subject matter I was studying in Higher Education Leadership. It taught me to be a thorough researcher. I learned to search for patterns in topics. I learned to evaluate, integrate, and synthesize information from knowledgeable experts in the field. This skill has served me well in my research and personal exploration to find the best nutritional dietary choices and other controversial alternative medical information. That research over the last four years supports the knowledge offered in this book. My personal health journey, and that of my husband, supports the knowledge in this book. This book offers an innovative and empowering alternative life style intervention strategy for a high quality of life as we age. Increased longevity does not mean better health and wellness as we age. We also need to engage in lifestyle changes that include proactive intervention life style changes and alternative decision-making. We must take responsibility for our health and wellness choices. There are multiple alternative health-related strategies that we must try in order to maintain our health and wellness, and this book outlines great choices to begin your journey. I heartily recommend this worthwhile book for all who will take the leap forward and become wealthier in their proactive healthy outlook and lifestyle choices.

Dr. Pat Sager Lane

Table of Contents

"You have to be lucky, but I made the best of things when bad things happened. I also ate prunes every single day."

— Morris Lensky, age 101

Chapter One

WHAT ACTUALLY HAPPENS WHEN YOU EAT?

> **"Food goes into your stomach (where juices are flowing), turns into paste, then the paste keeps on going. A tube, the intestine, is what food moves through. This food feeds your blood, which then feeds all of you."**
>
> **- Dr. Seuss.**

Have you ever really thought about what happens to food after you put it in your mouth? Do you think that once your hunger is satisfied that's the end of the game? You're in for a surprise. It's just the beginning. Once you have swallowed your food, all the work begins. It's like dropping something down a test tube. A long dark test tube, over 20 feet long, filled with powerful chemicals.

Good food makes you strong and healthy and gives you energy. However, before your body can use the food it has to change the food. Food is not automatically absorbed into the body for nourishment. It has to work to do that. Think of your body as your employee. You can either give that employee the ideal working conditions to accomplish his tasks and help you prosper (be healthy, happy, beautiful and vibrant), or you can load that employee down with, say, pens that don't write, phones that don't ring, computer software with viruses and lights that won't go on, and then yell and scream all day that he's not doing his job. You can't fire him because he is the only employee you have. So you scratch your head and stomp your feet and give him aspirins and drugs and supplements and wonder why the guy down the street has such a good employee and you got stuck with a dud.

We have news for you. Your employee is stupendous. His primary concern at all times is to keep you running; so you can't blame him if sometimes he takes those pens that don't write or phones that don't ring and shoves them into cubbyholes. He is operating under the theory of 'homeostasis', which means to keep internal balance at all costs. You're the one who is slacking. As the boss, it is up to you to help him be his optimal best. If you're starting late in life to think healthy, you may have years of poor living habits, poor choices, stress and fatigue to overcome while you retrain your employee to be a superstar...but you can do it and we're here to help you.

Your Digestive Process

To healers throughout the ages, most diseases begin and end with our food (whether it is physical food, mental food or spiritual food). For right now, we're just going to talk about physical food. We are taking extra time with the following explanations because it is vital to your health that you understand your body's digestive process. It is your equipment. You have to know how it works. You've probably spent more time learning your cell phone or ipad. Once you understand this, everything else we tell you will make perfect sense and you will be more willing to comply. When you comply, you will be healthy, you will tell all your family and friends, they will be healthy, we will have helped, WE will be happy. So please don't skip this part. There will be a test at the end of the chapter. By the way, your digestive system is commonly referred to as "your gut".

Digestion is the key to health. The act of digestion chemically changes the foods we eat into substances that can pass into the blood stream, circulate through the body, and feed our cells and organs. Every organ you have. Therefore, when you change the food you eat, you are digesting it. You are breaking it up into millions of very tiny pieces so you can use it. Our body (our employee) uses these nutritional substances for fuel, for repair, for rejuvenation and rebuilding, and to conduct an awesome symphony of biochemistry that scientists still do not fully understand, although we know just enough to stay healthy.

Chew

Beginning with your saliva, your body breaks down the food you eat into a series of different enzymes at several "stations" as it travels from your mouth to your stomach to your small intestines, to your large intestines, and then out the chute. Sometimes your body produces saliva before you even take a bite! That is how ready your body is to get the job done.

Did you know that 80% of our immune system is located in the gut and primarily depends on the bacteria that live there? Researchers have discovered that a gene that is essential for producing critical immune cells in your gut, responds to the food you eat—specifically leafy green vegetables.

An enzyme called ptyalin secreted by the salivary glands starts the job in your mouth to convert insoluble starches into simple sugars. If this is not done, (from lack of proper chewing) your body cannot extract the energy in your food and undigested starches pass through the stomach and into the intestines where they create a huge burden for your body by fermenting (and creating gas). This leaves a bigger mess for your liver to clean up. Just take a little cracker and chew it over and over.... It will practically dissolve in your mouth. That's ptyalin. One of the basic recommendations in Chinese Medicine is to chew your food 35 times. It is the easiest habit for weight loss you can imagine. So chew, chew, and chew. Repeat as you chew....the Power of ptyalin... the Power of ptyalin....the Power of ptyalin...

Once your nicely chewed food reaches your stomach, your stomach muscles continuously churn the food like the agitator in your washing machine. This forms a kind of ball in the stomach (called a bolus) which mixes with more digestive fluids such as hydrochloric acid and pepsin and is broken down into water-soluble amino acids. A completely different enzyme called lipase breaks down fatty foods. At this point, any starch that was not converted to sugar in your mouth is on its own, since the stomach's acidity virtually deactivates ptyalin (and ptyalin was the enzyme used to break down carbohydrates). See why Mom told us to chew?

The objective of digestion is taking insoluble foods and making them into water-soluble substances so they can pass into the blood stream and be used. Amino acids are soluble. Therefore, your body attempts to use the enzymes to break down the proteins to separate them into individual amino acids. Viola. With sufficient churning in the stomach over a few hours combined with the proper enzymes your proteins can be decomposed into amino acids that surf through your blood stream and are rebuilt into whatever the body needs for health.

EXCEPT when protein chains are heated (as with cooked meat and fish). Then the enzymes cannot attach themselves and the job can't get done. This is a big glitch. Cooked proteins are comparatively indigestible no matter what your body does. We know you don't want to hear this. Sad story, but true. Do not despair. If you eat meat, then just eat it in moderation... and not every day. You will just have to work a little harder at the elimination process down the road. We'll tell you how.

Heartburn: In some people, the contents of the stomach seep back up into the esophagus or lower gullet. This causes inflammation and pain in the chest where the acid attacks the gullet lining. The pain is known as heartburn. Between the stomach and the duodenum (upper part of your small intestine closest to the stomach) there is a muscle called the sphincter. When the sphincter relaxes, it opens and a small amount of food is squeezed into the duodenum, just as toothpaste moves out of the tube when the cap is off. After a small amount of food leaves the stomach, the sphincter quickly closes, sealing off the passageway. The rest of the food remains in the stomach until the duodenum is ready to receive it. This removal of food from the stomach prevents food from filling the stomach and inching up into the lower part of the esophagus. Because the gastric juices in the stomach are acid, an overflow could damage the tissue of the esophagus and cause this burning pain we call heartburn.

As if this wasn't bad enough, the stomach is considered 'your second brain' with 100 million nerve cells embedded in the lining called the enteric nervous system, which are influenced by your thoughts (and vice versa). Listen to your gut. Stress can inhibit digestive enzymes by telling your stomach to produce inflammatory chemicals; making otherwise digestible foods (starches, sugars, uncooked proteins) become indigestible. This is why, when you're upset, you get a stomach ache. Ever hear the phrase "Just the thought of it makes me sick"? In our Energetic Body chapter, we'll give you ways to keep your thoughts and emotions on track for optimal digestion.

The stomach can hold food from your last meal for hours. It slowly releases partially digested food into the next part of the digestive system, the small intestine, a little at a time. Any food that is too big for the small intestine stays in the stomach longer where the acid and pepsin continue to break it down further. Food should take no more than 48 hours from the stomach to ejection.

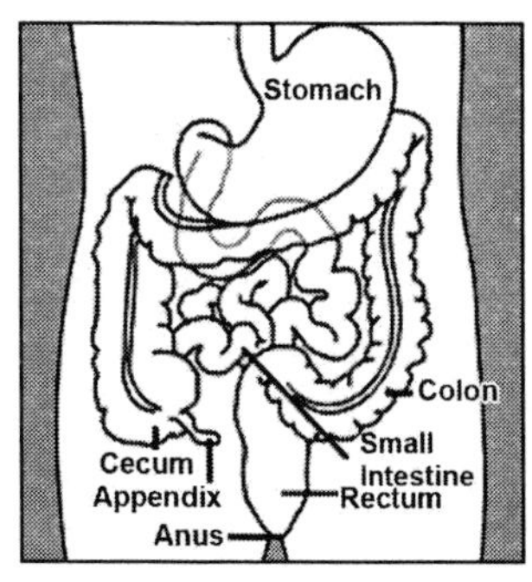

Now that we have broken up the food into millions of tiny pieces, we have to break it up even smaller. This happens in the intestines. Even though many people call their abdomen, or belly, their stomach, most of the

Helpful Hint: If you are "Bulky" right under your breasts you may be having difficulty digesting in your small intestines

abdomen is made up of the small and large intestines.

There are two intestines in your body – the small and the large. Really, they are just one long tube all coiled up inside of you. This tube is over 20 feet long and most of it is your small intestine, which is narrow (about one inch). That's why it's called the "small" intestine. Even though if you took it out and stood it up it would tower above your large intestines. The last 5 feet are wider and called the large intestine.

The small intestine is where most of the digestion and absorption of nutrients takes place. Food coming from the stomach mixes with enzymes and fluids coming from the pancreas and liver. These enzymes and fluids break up the food into molecules while neutralizing stomach acids. These molecules are the basic building blocks of our nutrition: amino acids, sugars, fatty acids, vitamins and minerals.

On the inside wall of the small intestine are thousands of very tiny, finger-like folds called villi. The villi have special channels, or tunnels, that allow the nutrients to leave the small intestine and enter the bloodstream. When the food we eat exits the small intestine, there is nothing left but water, some minerals, and material we can't digest, such as fiber.

The molecules then pass into tiny blood vessels and lymph vessels in the walls of the small intestine and move into your blood. Your blood then carries these molecules to every part of your body.

The part of the food that is not digested in the small intestine is then squeezed into the large intestine. From here water molecules pass into the bloodstream. The food you cannot use is stored in the large intestine and then eliminated through your bowel movements.

5 Steps of Digestion

As your meal travels though the gut, different enzymes break town different types of food. For example, only carbohydrates are broken down in the mouth. Carbohydrates and proteins are broken down in the stomach, while fats are mainly broken down in the small intestine.

Mouth: Approximately 1 minute or chewing 36 times to fully break down.

Esophagus: 5 - 10 seconds

Stomach: 1 - 3 hours

Small Intestine: 1 - 6 hours

Large Intestine: 12-36 hours

The Price of Gas

When undigested starches reach the small intestine, they are fermented by yeasts, which are part of the natural flora of your digestive system. The by-products of this fermentation are only slightly toxic but they do produce gas, which

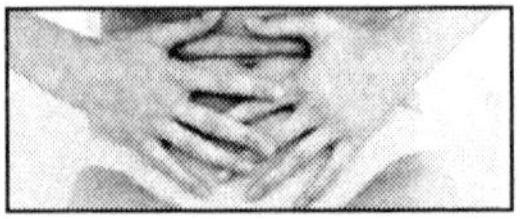

is odorless. You may feel an uncomfortable bloating. If you are healthy, it can take years and years of starch fermentation toxins to produce any disease in your body. The smart thing to do is to take steps to be sure that your starches are thoroughly digested.

Undigested proteins, on the other hand, are not fermented by yeast. While these proteins putrefy in the intestine, anaerobic bacteria attack them and a foul-smelling gas is produced. Many of the waste products of anaerobic putrefaction are highly toxic. These highly toxic waste products are absorbed through the small or large intestines and irritate those mucus membranes, where they can contribute to or cause cancer of the colon.

Additionally, these undigested proteins greatly compromise the functioning of your large intestine causing constipation. As far as your body is concerned, when it retains waste products in the large intestines way past the time that it should have exited you have constipation. Constipation causes harmful waste products of its own! Think of rush hour traffic getting really jammed up on the highway. People sitting in their cars for hours, then days, start throwing things out the window... the exhaust fumes cloud the skies, water and oil leak all over the highway. It's a mess.

Undigested food gradually coats the large intestines and putrefies further, becoming harder and narrowing the passage. These toxins can then move into the bloodstream and overwhelm our liver and kidneys until they are in a constant state of survival attempting to detoxify us. This causes malfunction of these organs as well, making us age faster and challenging hospitals and doctor offices to figure out our fascinating symptoms.

We are not done yet – there is more. When we ingest food substances that contain toxic dyes, chemicals, preservatives or genetically modified components, we're loading our body up with substances that it has no idea how to handle. This is sort of like piling a bunch of bricks on top of your employee.

Here is what happens: The toxins accumulate if we don't purge them immediately (which, by the way, we hardly ever do). First, they appear to us in liquid form. If they are not eliminated from our body, they are automatically and gradually dehydrated or crystallized. Then they are deposited in every available space throughout our cells, glands and organs. This is homeostasis at its finest! When there's just no place left to deposit them, nature reverses the action and slowly dissolves the crystallized and dehydrated material bringing it back to liquid form...because only in a fluid or semi fluid form can we eliminate our toxins. By this time, we have a major illness on our hands and our organs are clogged, overworked, and very inefficient. We grind to a halt. We develop any one of a dozen major diseases, from arthritis to renal failure.

We hope you can see at this point what this all means to your body. Foods that are not fully digested saddle your body with a heavy toxic weight and create havoc, greatly shortening your life span. Foods that contain toxins slow down and damage your system. We haven't even touched on the toxins that you drink, breathe, smell, put on your skin, or THINK (yes... we said think).

Additionally, 80% of your immune system is located in the gut and primarily depends on the bacteria that live there. In fact, a gene that is essential for producing critical immune cells in your gut responds to the food you eat (specifically, green leafy vegetables). What does this mean? It means that poor digestion can lead to repeated colds, flus, allergies, and inflammation.

A great book for your library is "What's your Poo Telling You?" along with its companion book, "What's My Pee Telling Me?", by Josh Richman and Anish Sheth. You can analyze your eliminations and get a better idea of what is happening on that digestive highway.

Everything we tell you from this point on is meant to optimize your digestive process so that your body works efficiently to provide you with optimal health, happiness and beauty. Plain and simple - effortless health. So, we are asking you: Do you have the guts to get healthy?

Liver, Gallbladder and Pancreas

Although not located directly in the digestive tract, this thankless trio is an integral part of our digestive system. The liver makes bile that passes to a small storage bag called the gallbladder. The liver produces two pints of bile every day and the gallbladder stores it. After the stomach releases its contents into the intestines, the gallbladder squirts bile down the tubes to help digest the food.

Your pretty pink pancreas, situated alongside the stomach with the small intestine looping around it, makes digestive juices that flow though a duct into the small intestine. These juices help neutralize the stomach acid so it doesn't burn the gut. They also contain enzymes that help to break down protein, starch and fat in food so they can be absorbed. Your pancreas also produces insulin and glucagon, which help to control the blood's level of the sugar glucose, the body's main source of energy. Too much or too little sugar can cause a myriad of problems in your body, including diabetes.

Your wedge shaped, workaholic organ, the liver, is situated in the center of your core to the right of your midline. Like a huge, hectic kitchen, it processes raw ingredients brought in by your blood from the stomach and intestines. At this point, it cleans the blood from any toxins that may have been absorbed by the small intestines. Therefore, when you ingest toxins, you are making more work for your body right down the line. The liver whips up bile, and stores sugar and nutrients. The liver is constantly working itself into a frenzy, managing over 500 functions, and heating up the entire body in the process.

The liver is a wizard at sorting good things from bad. Poisons are whisked away while medicines are broken down and activated so they can get to work in the body. Once toxins are neutralized, we toss some out with the bile. The rest go in the blood to the kidneys to be filtered out of the body. In a healthy adult, the liver weighs an average of 3 to 4 pounds. It has the amazing ability to repair itself and even regrow parts of itself if it is injured.

Chemical reaction units called enzymes do the liver's main jobs.

The Kidneys

While your blood is delivering nutrients around the body, it also takes the time to collect waste and unwanted products from cells and tissues. It then rids itself of these wastes via the urinary system. The urinary system consists of two kidneys located at the back of the upper abdomen, with tubes that carry the urine down to the bladder.

Every 10 minutes all of your body's blood passes through the kidneys where it is filtered. This means that your blood is filtered about 150 times a day. Filtered urine passes into the bladder, which can hold from one to two pints. When kidneys become diseased or fail, the blood cannot be filtered properly. Toxic blood is then recirculated throughout the body and waste builds up everywhere. Being sufficiently hydrated with plenty of water and good liquids helps your natural filtering process. Drink your water and eat your fruits and vegetables, which have very high water content!

STEPS TO INTEGRATE INTO YOUR DAILY HABITS

- Get in the habit of chewing thoroughly
- Pay attention to how you feel after each meal
- Notice if your stomach becomes distended, or if you have gas

SELF-TEST FOR CHAPTER ONE

1. What is homeostasis?

a. Staying home on holidays
b. Your body's effort to keep you running and balanced no matter what
c. A standing man

2. What is the key to health?

a. Herbs
b. Good dishes
c. Digestion

3. Where does digestion first begin?

a. In the supermarket
b. In the oven
c. In your mouth

4. What are digestive enzymes?

a. A new line of clothing for tennis players
b. A corner café in New Orleans
c. Enzymes that break down food into their smaller building blocks in order to facilitate their absorption by the body.

5. What happens to undigested food?

a. It can give you gas
b. You won't be able to absorb the nutrients
c. The food coats the large intestines
d. All of the above

6. What is a toxin?

a. A poisonous, usually unstable compound
b. A German taxicab
c. A type of sit-com.

7. Where do toxins go in your body?

a. To your large intestines
b. To your organs
c. To all your cells and joints
d. All of the above

8. How do your organs, muscles, bones, nerves and cells get nutrients?

a. Through singing
b. Through your blood
c. Through digestion
d. Both b and c

9. How many functions does your liver have?

a. One: to process my beers
b. 15
c. 50
d. 500

10. Foul smelling gas is caused by:

a. An old car
b. Undigested carbohydrates
c. Undigested proteins
d. All of the above.

"He who has health, has hope;
and he who has hope, has everything."

— Thomas Carlyle

Chapter Two

FOODS TO AVOID

Are you ready? Take a deep breath. You can do this. Now that you understand what your body is desperately trying to do for you, you need to give it all the support you can muster.

> **To keep the body in good health is a duty; Otherwise, we shall not be able to keep our mind strong and clear.**
> **- Buddha**

Understand that when you eat toxic substances such as chemicals and preservatives, or foods your body thinks it is allergic to; or if you don't eliminate by-products in a timely manner, your body will become inflamed. So what? Inflammation is a dangerous game. It is the body's attempt at self-protection. Its objective is to remove harmful stimuli, irritants, pathogens, even damaged cells, and begin the healing process. It quickly gives immune cells and key nutrients their marching orders to reach the site of the injury or invasion in order to bring peace to the area. These fighter cells get there through increased blood flow causing the swelling, warmth, redness and sometimes pain.

The problem is, when we are in a constant state of inflammation, the healing process can never begin and the immune system starts going haywire and attacking everything - even healthy cells. It never shuts off, constantly producing immune cells that can do permanent damage and lead to cancer, heart disease, arthritis, etc. It can be self-perpetuating, inflammation, causing more inflammation, and then causing more inflammation, until you have an autoimmune disease. Studies show that if celiac disease is not addressed (the body's allergy to wheat) it can trigger Multiple sclerosis, ALS, Fibromyalgia, Crohn's, Cancer and Alzheimer's among many other autoimmune diseases.

The cause of chronic inflammation varies, but almost invariably comes down to the food we eat and the lifestyle we choose. We need proper sleep, proper diet, proper exercise and mindfulness to keep our bodies at peace.

Start out avoiding any foods that are genetically modified or engineered. The first GMOs were quietly introduced into our food supply in 1996. Every day new studies come out showing the danger of genetically modified food. There are many clinical studies showing statistics of the rise of many diseases since GMOs were introduced into our food supply. Corn is genetically engineered with a pesticide (Bt) right in the seed, so that when insects try to eat the corn their stomachs explode. That makes you kind of wonder what it's doing to you, right? The inflammation caused by GMOs is now being linked to Parkinson's, Dementia, Leaky Gut syndrome, Diabetes, Thyroid disorder, and more. Genetically modified foods are programmed with not only pesticides, but with the genes of other plants (and sometimes even animals) for a higher growth/less risk/more profit formula for the corporations. Viruses and bacteria are used in the modification for optimal saturation and depth. For more information about genetically modified foods, check out these web sites:

www.responsibletechnology.org

www.undergroundhealth.com

www.nongmoshoppingguide.com/tips-for-avoiding-gmos.html

You can also watch an incredibly informative video for free on *YouTube* called Genetic Roulette. Please do. Please educate yourself. Your health and the health of those you love depend on it. Your digestive system is YOUR equipment. Treat it as well as you treat your car, your computer, your cell phone.

A simple way to avoid genetically modified foods is to buy organic. Organic farmers are prohibited from using GMO seeds.

The top 7 genetically modified crops (that you will want to avoid) are as follows:

Corn: (88% grown in the USA) is genetically modified) Buy only organic corn on the cob. However, realize that corn, corn oil, cornstarch, and at least a dozen different derivatives are in processed foods.

Soy: (93% is genetically modified) Soy is a staple in processed foods and goes under various names including: hydrogenated oils, lecithin, emulsifiers, tocopherol (a vitamin E supplement) and proteins. Isolated soy proteins can actually mimic estrogen cell receptors and disrupt your hormones! Now that should make you mad.

Cottonseed: (94% of cotton grown in the USA is genetically modified) cottonseed, made from GMO cotton, is used in vegetable oil, margarine, frying foods (think potato chips).

Alfalfa: The fourth largest crop to be GMO, is fed to dairy cows, the source of milk, butter, yogurt, meat and much, much more.

Papaya: 75% of Hawaiian papaya is genetically modified.

Canola: 90% of US canola crop is genetically modified. Canola is oil, and you will find it as an ingredient in many processed foods.

Sugar Beets: 54% of sugar sold in America comes from sugar beets – and 90% of that is genetically modified.

It is not the intent of this book to cover all that needs to be said on genetically modified foods, so please research further.

We are going to name a few other standout habits that need to be eliminated if you want to experience your optimal energy and health. To make it easier on yourself when you read the ingredients here is a rule of thumb to go by:

1. If it has more than five ingredients that should put up a red flag for you.
2. If there are ingredients that you can't pronounce... stick up another red
3. If you see any of the top seven GMO crops, refined sugar, white flour, bleached flour, anything that says "artificial", or hydrogenated oil... pretend both red flags just hit you on the head.

Artificial Sweeteners should be avoided at all costs. So this, of course, means all sodas. Some web sites to understand why are: http://verdavivo.wordpress.com/2009/02/12/14-reasons-not-to-drink-soda/

Tobacco and Alcohol: This goes without saying – but we're saying it anyway. If you want to be on the road to a healthier lifestyle, you will have to give these two little demons up. Eventually. However, don't let them stop you... starting to eat healthy first gives you that fresh, clean, energetic feeling so that you will WANT to give these up. Eventually.

Fried foods and processed foods are a no-no. Yes. That's what we said. They are carcinogenic. This means most cold cuts, too. Therefore, you'll have to reinvent your sandwich.

Coffee is one of the most toxic substances on the planet because of how it is sprayed and processed. If you can't give it up then at least only drink organic coffee. For a while, anyway. Then give it up. Some people we know only use coffee for enemas!

White Flour Products: Try to lessen your intake of white flour products. They are very mucus forming. In oriental medicine mucus is dampness. Dampness leads to tumors. Mix it with heat in the body (inflammation) and it leads to cancer. So let's keep dampness at a minimum from the start.

Cow's milk... especially reduced fat or low fat. Cows are injected with GM bovine growth hormone, which has been condemned by the American Public Health Association, American Nurses Association, and numerous others due to its potential for increasing cancer risk. Look for labels stating No rBGH, rBST, or artificial hormones. Unless your milk is organic, the cow that it came from is fed GMO corn, soy and alfalfa. It's in their blood. It's in their milk. You would be doing yourself a big favor to avoid all cows' milk. Don't worry, we list several delicious milks for you to drink from other sources under FOODS TO EAT that are actually good for you and far surpass the taste of drugged cow's milk.

Sodas: They are loaded with chemicals and artificial sweeteners, the most dangerous being aspartame. Many sodas that advertise "natural sweeteners" and have sugar on their labels use genetically modified sugar from sugar beets. That is an ingredient on our "avoid" list. There is not one good thing in soda. Stay away from it. Don't worry; we're going to give you things to drink that are just as tasty AND good for you!

So now, you're getting the picture of why we are currently having an "organic craze". Certified organic products cannot INTENTIONALLY include any GMO ingredients. Buy products labeled "100% organic" if only to avoid GMOs. "Made with Organic ingredients" means only 70% of the product is organic. You can be doubly sure a product is safe if it is organic AND has a Non-GMO Project Verified Seal on it. If your product is not labeled organic or verified non-GMO, then avoid those products made with the top 7 genetically modified crops.

When animal products are sold or labeled as organically produced it means they are not given any kind of antibiotics, or growth hormones, are only fed with organic feed, and are not administered any type of medication aside from vaccinations or to treat an illness

Fruits and vegetables that are labeled and sold as organic are grown without using most pesticides or fertilizers with synthetic ingredients, there is no irradiation treatment; seeds and transplants are chemical-free, and the fertilizer is natural. This means a lot less chemicals in your body and a lot more antioxidants and nutrients.

If you cannot make your entire diet organic, then here is a list called ***The Dirty Dozen*** (foods with the highest pesticide residue). This list is from the Environmental Working Group. www.environmentalworkinggroup.org You will want to make THESE organic in your diet:

Apples	Celery	Cherry Tomatoes
Cucumbers	Grapes	Hot Peppers
Nectarines	Peaches	Potatoes
Strawberries	Spinach	Sweet Bell Peppers

In addition, here is a list of ***THE CLEAN FOURTEEN***. These foods have the least amount of pesticides, so eating non organic is not such a risk to your health. You may find a "Clean Fifteen" list on the internet. Our list is only fourteen long because we have excluded corn - one of the topmost genetically modified foods of today.

Asparagus	Avocado	Cabbage
Cantaloupe	Sweet Potatoes	Eggplant
Grapefruit	Kiwi	Mango
Watermelon	Mushrooms	Onions
Pineapple	Sweet Peas	

Keep it simple so you don't stress out. There are actually apps for your Smartphone now that you can refer to while you are at the grocery store. Keep your diet fresh and whole. Steer clear of most boxes and cans. Frozen fruit and vegetables are fine, but again, read the ingredients. Some of those large packaged frozen meals are filled with much more then you see on the pretty picture on the cover. Do not worry...there's lots and lots of great tasting food left to eat!

A Word about GLUTEN. We would be doing you a grave injustice if we didn't outline to you how dangerous gluten can be for you if you are sensitive to it. Over the past 50 years, this condition has increased to the unbelievable rate of 1 in every 100 people. In addition, given the problems in diagnosing, the statistics may be even higher than that. The problem is that there is not yet a clear-cut inexpensive test to see if you are sensitive to it.

What is gluten? Gluten is a protein made up of the peptides gliadin and glutenin and is found in many grains such as wheat, semolina, spelt, kamut, rye and barley. (Don't worry - there is now a gluten free beer!) It is also used as a stabilizing agent in many processed foods and condiments.

Many people ask why previous generations never worried about wheat. The wheat you are eating today is not the same grain that your parents (or even you) consumed in the past. It has been significantly hybridized and deamidated in order for it to be more bug-resistant, drought-resistant and faster growing. There is now a multitude of new proteins in our wheat that our bodies are not recognizing as friendly. The hybridization of wheat has created a "new wheat" that appears to cause inflammation in the body - especially to the brain and nervous system. Read Dr. Perlmutter's ground breaking book, THE GRAIN BRAIN if you really want to blow your mind.

The immune response many people are having to wheat appears to be a major driver of chronic inflammation, intestinal permeability (leaky gut) and autoimmunity. Think arthritis, fibromyalgia, lupus, digestive disorders, and thyroid dysfunction.

As more doctors are beginning to recognize the symptoms of gluten intolerance, it is being diagnosed with more efficiency each day. There really is not much difference between gluten sensitivity and celiac disease other than the intensity of the reaction. Many people with gluten sensitivity do not have intestinal problems, but rather the gluten can affect other tissues such as in the brain, thyroid, joints, bones, heart, liver, pancreas, reproductive organs and the nervous system. Still want that sandwich?

Here is an overview of what happens in your stomach when you eat gluten:

Everything you eat that contains gluten has an identical effect on your digestive system. When your donut reaches your intestines, it is broken down so the proteins can be absorbed. In those with gluten sensitivity, the protein is identified as a dangerous substance and your body produces antibodies to attack it. When this happens, the microvillus in your gut is compromised. The microvilli erode, you can no longer absorb nutrients as you should, and the walls of your intestines become leaky. This can cause symptoms such as bloating, constipation, diarrhea, weight loss, weight gain, fat malabsorbtion and malnutrition, iron deficiency or anemia and low vitamin D.

That's not all this little donut can do. A leaky gut allows toxins, microbes undigested food particles and antibodies to escape from your intestines and run wild throughout your body surfing through your bloodstream.

These rogue antibodies now end up attacking other organs and systems from the skin to the thyroid to the brain. That's why gluten intolerance is frequently paired with autoimmune conditions. Gluten intolerance untreated also causes many other food allergies, as your system is primed for attack on a continual basis. Suddenly you find yourself with a runny nose when you eat tomatoes or an itchy throat whenever you have rice, maybe those almonds you love start giving you a headache. If your gut is compromised, allergies can pop up anytime with anything. Sometimes, you have no digestive symptoms at all... and this is the scariest... because sometimes your autoimmune response takes place in the blood brain barrier and you find your memory is not what it used to be. Alternatively, you're moody. (Did you get that book yet? *GRAIN BRAIN* by Dr. Perlmutter!)

The only difference between celiac disease and gluten sensitivity is the severity of instant reaction. Both cause long term inflammation in the body when wheat or gluten is consumed.

There are three stages of autoimmunity and your body travels through them like a stealth bomber.

First Stage: Silent autoimmunity. We have antibodies but no symptoms. Antibodies show up well ahead of the dysfunction and you can predict which tissue is tagged for future dysfunction. It is a predictive diagnostic concept to be tested for antibodies. Many physicians who practice functional blood chemistry analysis will test your blood for certain antibodies.

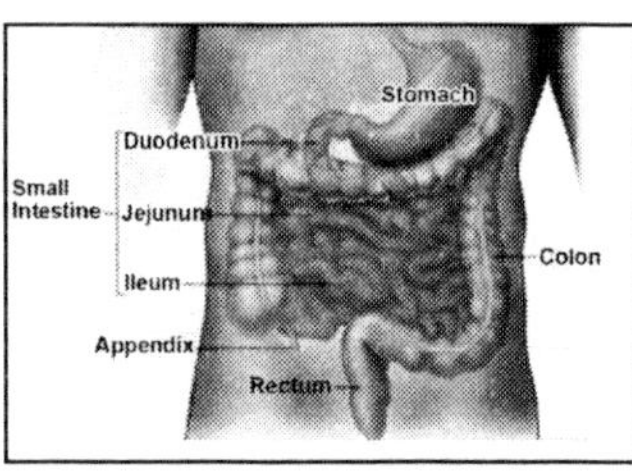

Second Stage: Reactive autoimmunity. We have antibodies plus symptoms but have not yet lost extreme amounts of tissue.

Third Stage: Autoimmunity Disease. We have antibodies plus the disease and major loss of tissue. (There are as many as 80 types of autoimmune diseases, from lupus to rheumatoid arthritis. Many have the same symptoms, which makes them hard to diagnose.)

If you have any allergies at all, give up gluten. If you have any food allergies at all, give up gluten. If you have any autoimmune diseases, give up gluten. If you have arthritis or diabetes, give up gluten. Are you getting this? Give up gluten. It's not hard.

We know that by now you are frozen with fear. How will I eat? How will I feed my family? What's left? Believe us, there is plenty. Once you get in the swing of things and start dropping pounds, feeling more energetic, happier, thinking clearer, and yes – even watching your children behave better, you will wonder how you ever survived eating what you eat right now.

Check out www.greenmedinfo.com for a steady stream of current health articles on gluten, GMOs and other toxins to our health.

Books:

Against the Grain by Jax Peters Lowell

The Gluten-Free Bible by Jax Peters Lowell

The Grain Brain by Dr. Perlmutter

The No-Grain Diet by Dr Mercola

Steps to integrate into your daily habits

- Start buying more and more organic foods to avoid GMOs
- Use fresh fruit and vegetables and whole grains
- Go gluten free for one month. When you see a difference – don't go back.
- Check ingredients – get rid of one GMO ingredient per week from top 7 list (for example – no more items with cottonseed oil... then no more items with canola oil, etc.)

SELF TEST FOR CHAPTER TWO

1. What is a Genetically Modified food?

a. food that has been put in a blender

b. food that has had the addition of genetic material from other organisms through molecular techniques

c. food that has graduated college.

2. What is Bt-corn, or Bt. Potatoes or Bt cotton?

a. the plants are able to produce pesticides inside themselves

b. the plants themselves are toxic

c. both a and b

3. The highest pesticide residue is found on?

a. Apples

b. Celery

c. Strawberries

d. All three (and more)

4. People may be sensitive to gluten because

a. They can't cook.

b. They eat too much

c. Wheat has been hybridized and deamidated in recent years and contains more proteins now that are harmful to our bodies.

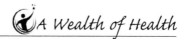

5. If you are sensitive to gluten it can

a. Cause the walls of your intestines to weaken and allow toxins in the body.

b. Cause bloating, constipation, weight gain, anemia, autoimmunity and more

c. Cause you to be unable to absorb nutrients

d. All of the above

6. What is autoimmunity.

a. Your body attacks its own cells and tissues

b. A yearly renewal to a local club

c. A community car rental business

7. Why is the first stage of autoimmunity so dangerous?

a. Because a lot of people don't bring the cars back.

b. If you don't renew you won't get into the club

c. Because there are no symptoms – and yet damage is still being done continuously.

"Do what you have to do.
Don't analyze it, just do it."

— Johanna Zurndorfer, age 97

SO WHAT CAN I EAT?

Now the fun part! We get to tell you about all the delicious, nutritious foods there are left on the table. We want to make sure we have balance. The trick is to pick a variety of foods from each category. Start out simply. Experiment. This is a learning process, but it is not hard. In fact, it can be fun. Whatever we eat, good or bad, is either a protein, carbohydrate or a fat. These macronutrients are essential for health and our diet needs to include all three categories. All protein, carbohydrates and fats have calories.All of our food sources also contain micronutrients, which are vitamins, minerals and phytochemicals. They are calorie-free. Therefore, we will start with the macronutrients.

Fats. There are good and bad fats. The good fats are Omega 3, Omega 6, polyunsaturated fats, Monounsaturated (Omega 9) fatty acids, CLA and healthy saturated fats found in raw dairy products and coconut. All the above-mentioned fats are found in a wide variety of foods including:

Salmon	Olives	Chia seeds
Tuna	Avocado	Borage Seeds
Lamb	Macadamia nuts	Flaxseeds
Goat Meat	Walnuts	Sunflower seeds

Salmon also has protein in it... so there is a food that provides protein along with good fats. The same holds true for tuna or lamb. In fact, as you learn, you will find that whole, natural foods generally provide two or three essential elements for health, bite for bite.

Protein: This is the major building block for muscles, blood, skin, hair, nails and the internal organs including the heart and the brain. It increases stamina and supports the immune system. It controls bodily functions such as growth and metabolism and is needed for hormone formation. So, you see, proteins do a lot of work in the body. However, recent studies are showing that we really do not need as much protein as we think we do. Additionally, although lean beef, turkey and chicken contain high amounts of protein, as does salmon, tuna and halibut, our protein does not have to come from animal flesh, as we are so often led to believe.

Other sources of protein:

- Raw milk or kefir
- Raw cheese from grass fed cows
- Wheatgrass juice
- Microalges (spirulina, chlorella and AFA)
- Leafy greens such as spinach or kale and their juices
- Sesame seeds
- Avocados
- Almonds
- Eggs, which should be only from organic and preferably local sources
- Raw coconut cream

Carbohydrates: You can get most every carbohydrate you need from your fruits and vegetables. For that extra something-something on the side at dinner, try these gluten-free whole grains:

- **Amaranth** is higher in protein than most other grains. It has a peppery flavor.
- **Millet** can be used in recipes that call for rice. It is a good source of antioxidants.
- **Quinoa** A great source of protein, fiber, B vitamins and iron. You can prepare it a week in advance and it can be used in soups and salads.
- **Brown Rice** is always yummy if you don't want to try anything new!

You can make dozens and dozens of healthy, delicious, nutritious meals from what we have listed. However, we are not done. We will provide you with a variety of little secrets and food tables to help you constantly choose the best foods and get the most from each and every bite.

To be the healthiest you can be, you will want to familiarize yourself with the micronutrient content in your food. Eating foods that have a high density of micronutrients have a far-reaching positive impact on human cell function and the immune system; promoting self-healing mechanisms throughout your body.

On the following page is a handy table of nutrient density scores from drfurhman.com. Dr. Fuhrman is the author of *Eat to Live*.

In addition to micronutrients, you may also want to review which foods have the highest enzyme content. Remember we spoke about enzymes back when we explained the digestive process? Metabolic enzymes produced by the pancreas perform a wide variety of functions. Breathing, eating, sleeping, digestion, absorption of nutrients, energy growth, circulation and more, all depend on metabolic enzymes. Some digestive enzymes are found in the mouth and the digestive tract where they aid in the digestion of food. (Remember ptyalin?) Well, did you know there are some foods that contain their own enzymes? Even more enzymes can be found in raw foods and help you initiate the process of digestion in the mouth and stomach. Wouldn't that be nice? Lessening your workload!

Dr. Furhman's Table of Nutrient Density Scores					
Kale	1000	Cantaloupe	100	Skim Milk	36
Collards	1000	Kidney Beans	100	Walnuts	34
Bok Choy	824	Sweet Potato	83	Grapes	31
Spinach	739	Black Beans	83	White Potato	31
Broccoli Rabe	715	Sunflower Seeds	78	Banana	30
Chinese/Napa Cabbage	704	Apple	76	Cashews	27
Brussel Sprouts	672	Peach	73	Chicken Breast	27
Swiss Chard	670	Green Peas	70	Eggs	27
Arugula	559	Cherries	68	Peanut Butter	26
Cabbage	481	Flax Seeds	65	Whole Wheat Bread	25
Romaine Lettuce	389	Pineapple	64	Feta Cheese	21
Broccoli	376	Chick Peas	57	Whole Milk	20
Carrot Juice	344	Oatmeal	53	Ground Beef	20
Cauliflower	295	Pumpkin Seeds	52	White Pasta	18
Green Peppers	258	Mango	51	White Bread	18
Artichoke	244	Cucumber	50	Apple Juice	16
Carrots	240	Soybeans	48	Swiss Cheese	15
Asparagus	234	Pistachio Nuts	48	Low Fat Yogurt	14
Strawberries	212	Corn	44	Potato Chips	11
Pomegranate Juice	193	Brown Rice	41	American Cheese	10
Tomato	164	Salmon	39	Vanilla Ice Cream	9
Blueberries	130	Almonds	38	French Fries	7
Iceberg Lettuce	110	Shrimp	38	Olive Oil	2
Orange	109	Avocado	37	Cola	1
Lentils	100	Tofu	37		

The above list of raw foods provides much more than just enzymes. Remember them when making a salad, or simply snacking. Not only will these foods keep your digestive system humming, they will fill you with dozens of living nutrients for optimal performance and energy.

Top Enzyme Foods:

- Raw cultured dairy yogurt and kefir from grass-fed cows have sixty known enzymes. Some of the enzymes are native to raw milk while others come from the beneficial bacteria growing in the milk. Because of the enzymes, this makes milk more digestible and frees up key minerals.
- Wild Salmon Ceviche, which is marinated in lemon or lime juice. This is loaded with pepsin, which are protein-digesting enzymes.
- Raw butter is a supreme source of lipases, fat-splitting enzymes that support our health in the areas of immune, brain and nervous system function.
- Raw sauerkraut contains naturally occurring enzymes that are beneficial to the digestive tract. Be sure to use raw, not processed, sauerkraut. Processed sauerkraut is processed with heat and made with vinegar.
- Avocados provide protein, healthy unsaturated fats and enzymes galore.
- Bananas are another enzyme rich food, but use caution, the more ripe they are the more enzymes are lost in the process. Try to eat them before they are too ripe.
- Pineapple is the main source of bromelain, a protein-digesting enzyme that supports healthy inflammation. Again, the less ripe the pineapple the more enzymes.

- Raw coconut kefir provides billions of probiotics and is loaded with enzymes and beneficial minerals such as potassium.

Now that we have listed so many delicious foods that you can mix, match, and experiment with, let's define them one step further so that you don't start eating too many foods that are a high acid content. We want our body to be more toward the alkaline state than the acidic in order to have the pH of gastric juices at an optimal level to break down the foods we eat. Health is all about digestion.

Let's separate our foods into two categories.... ACID and ALKALINE. Pretend you can see teams in your mind. When our body is in an alkaline state, it is better equipped to fight off diseases. Put that team in super hero suits. When our body is in an acid state, it attracts diseases. So put some evil flashy costumes on that team. It makes sense to increase your intake of alkaline foods while decreasing your intake of acidic foods. The rule of thumb is to strive for 80% alkaline foods and 20% acidic foods. Just do the best you can.

There are quite a few acid/alkaline charts circulating on the internet, in books and at health food stores. You may find differences among the charts, but the acid forming foods are consistently the same. Again, do the best you can. Don't stress out or expect perfection. It makes you acidic. Review the acid/alkaline chart on the next page and see if there are acidic foods on the list that you eat with any frequency. Gauge if your

Alkaline Forming Foods

VEGETABLES
Garlic
Asparagus
Fermented Veggies
Watercress
Beets
Broccoli
Brussel sprouts
Cabbage
Carrot
Cauliflower
Celery
Chard
Chlorella
Collard Greens
Cucumber
Eggplant
Kale
Kohlrabi
Lettuce
Mushrooms
Mustard Greens
Dulce
Dandelions
Edible Flowers
Onions
Parsnips (high glycemic)
Peas
Peppers
Pumpkin
Rutabaga
Sea Veggies
Spirulina
Sprouts
Squashes
Alfalfa
Barley Grass
Wheat Grass
Wild Greens
Nightshade Veggies

FRUITS
Apple
Apricot
Avocado
Banana (high glycemic)
Cantaloupe
Cherries
Currants
Dates/Figs
Grapes
Grapefruit
Lime
Honeydew Melon
Nectarine
Orange
Lemon
Peach
Pear
Pineapple
All Berries
Tangerine
Tomato
Tropical Fruits
Watermelon

PROTEIN
Eggs (poached)
Whey Protein Powder
Cottage Cheese
Chicken Breast
Yogurt
Almonds
Chestnuts
Tofu (fermented)
Flax Seeds
Pumpkin Seeds
Tempeh (fermented)
Squash Seeds
Sunflower Seeds
Millet
Sprouted Seeds
Nuts

OTHER
Apple Cider Vinegar
Bee Pollen
Lecithin Granules
Probiotic Cultures
Green Juices
Veggies Juices
Fresh Fruit Juice
Organic Milk (unpasteurized)
Mineral Water
Alkaline Antioxidant Water
Green Tea
Herbal Tea
Dandelion Tea
Ginseng Tea
Banchi Tea
Kombucha

SWEETENERS
Stevia
Ki Sweet

SPICES/ SEASONINGS
Cinnamon
Curry
Ginger
Mustard
Chili Pepper
Sea Salt
Miso
Tamari
All Herbs

ORIENTAL VEGETABLES
Maitake
Daikon
Dandelion Root
Shitake
Kombu
Reishi
Nori
Umeboshi
WakameSea Veggies

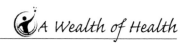

Acid Forming Foods

FATS & OILS
Avocado Oil
Canola Oil
Corn Oil
Hemp Seed Oil
Flax Oil
Lard
Olive Oil
Safflower Oil
Sesame Oil
Sunflower Oil
FRUITS
Cranberries
GRAINS
Rice Cakes
Wheat Cakes
Amaranth
Barley
Buckwheat
Corn
Oats (rolled)
Quinoa
Rice (all)
Rye
Spelt
Kamut
Wheat
Hemp Seed Flour
DAIRY
Cheese, Cow
Cheese, Goat
Cheese, Processed
Cheese, Sheep
Milk
Butter

NUTS & BUTTERS
Cashews
Brazil Nuts
Peanuts
Peanut Butter
Pecans
Tahini
Walnuts
ANIMAL PROTEIN
Beef
Carp
Clams
Fish
Lamb
Lobster
Mussels
Oyster
Pork
Rabbit
Salmon
Shrimp
Scallops
Tuna
Turkey
Venison
PASTA (WHITE)
Noodles
Macaroni
Spaghetti
OTHER
Distilled Vinegar
Wheat Germ
Potatoes

DRUGS & CHEMICALS
Aspartame
Chemicals
Drugs, Medicinal
Drugs, Psychedelic
Pesticides
Herbicides
ALCOHOL
Beer
Spirits
Hard Liquor
Wine
BEANS & LEGUMES
Black Beans
Chick Peas
Green Peas
Kidney Beans
Lentils
Lima Beans
Pinto Beans
Red Beans
Soy Beans
Soy Milk
White Beans
Rice Milk
Almond Milk

diet falls mostly on the acid or alkaline side by recognizing what you normally eat and where it falls on the chart. Now is the time to take stock of your daily eating habits and see what you can change to make yourself naturally more alkaline on a continuous basis.

"The body is a mirror of the mind."

— Unknown

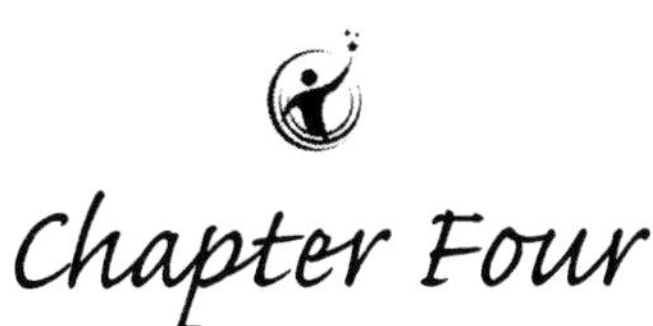

Chapter Four

CHEERS TO LIQUIDS

We can't just eat all day. We have to provide our body with liquids for hydration so our body-machine can operate at maximum efficiency. Being hydrated is also essential for losing weight and releasing toxins from our cells. Did you know that you couldn't lose weight if you are dehydrated? That alone should have you tipping the glass to your lips right now. Dehydration may also contribute to depression and pain.

Chinese Proverb: With true friends... even water drunk together is sweet enough.

So, what's to drink? Water is your best option here. If you get tired of drinking water, then add lemon, lime, or ginger to it.

All are additives that can boost your alkalinity and keep your motor nice and clean. It is very easy to purchase a large inexpensive container with a spout on it; fill it with good, clean, water; add lemon or lime, ginger, cucumbers, or any fruit you want; and, voila, you have a drinking beverage that is served at elitist spas.

Drink two glasses of lemon water right after waking up – helps activate internal organs and hydrate your body.

Drink 1 glass of water 30 minutes before a meal - helps digestion and hydration.

Drink 1 glass of water before taking a bath - helps lower blood pressure.

Drink one glass of water before going to bed - avoids stroke or heart attack, as well as nighttime leg cramps.

Minimum amount of water you should drink: Taking your weight and dividing it by two gives you the number of ounces to drink per day.

Sometimes Ursula adds zipfizz to her water, an energy supplement that she gets at Costco.Not that Ursula needs more energy! Please note that when she does occasionally use it, she uses only 1/3 of the tube in her water.

If you can, please stay away from bottled water. Typically, it is no healthier than tap water. Well water can be even worse. You can buy yourself a little hot/cold cooler and then refill the bottles at a trusted water site in your grocery. You can also get some good filter products for your tap at home. We have given you some links in Chapter 10 - Resources for that.

Drinking water continuously actually decreases fluid retention and helps your body remove cellular waste more efficiently. Do not drink water 20 minutes prior to or 20 minutes after your meal because it will dilute your digestive enzymes. (We spoke about digestive enzymes in Chapter 2).

There is presently controversy over the topic of drinking alkaline water all the time. The latest studies show that the benefits of detoxing and balancing your body with alkaline water only last a short time. If you drink alkaline water all the time, you are going to raise the alkalinity of your stomach, which will buffer your acidity and impair your ability to digest food. For more information on this topic visit articles.mercola.com and search alkaline or alkalized water.

However, we know that, short-term, alkaline water can provide benefits.

The human body creates acid, all day, every day, as a by-product of metabolism and stress! The American diet is extremely acidic, and combined with a stressful lifestyle, your body can easily manifest "acid overload."

Disorders such as acid reflux, high cholesterol, heart disease, excessive fat, and inflammatory related diseases such as allergies, arthritis, fibromyalgia, psoriasis, and even stroke are all related to low-grade metabolic acidosis.

Drinking alkaline water can help restore the pH in the body and reduce its acidity. (The pH scale measures how acidic a substance is and ranges from zero to 14.) The higher your pH, the healthier your body! Disease does not and cannot grow in an alkaline system. For example, cancer must have an acid base to survive and thrive. Cancer cannot grow in an alkaline system! In addition, alkaline water is negatively charged and an "antioxidant." Antioxidants reduce cellular and DNA damage caused by free radicals.

Alkaline water provides superior hydration and nutrition at the cellular level and detoxifies cells more efficiently than standard drinking water.

There are many ionized water systems from which to choose. So, just go on-line and compare water systems, prices and warranties.

Similar to raw food being 'living food', there is a type of water called 'living water.' Water that is clean, balanced and healthful, neither too acidic nor too alkaline is the best. Most of these waters are from mountain springs. If you would like to research more on this topic, www.findaspring.com would be a good place to start.

Depending on which day it is and what you were doing the night before, the right drink to balance you out and bounce you back can differ greatly. Luckily, we are extremists and can handle almost any situation. Read on to find the best drink for you to start the day.

Other great beverages that are either cleansing, nutritious, or both are:

Aloe Vera Liquid: Aloe contains nine minerals that interact to boost enzyme metabolic pathways. This increased enzyme activity ensures detoxification of wastes. It also stimulates the immune system functions and stimulates the production of white blood cells to help protect your body from disease. Additionally, it has anti-inflammatory properties that can heal internal wounds (think colitis and heartburn), help with pain, and increase water absorption and alleviate constipation. There are even studies that it helps with high cholesterol and hair loss. Because of the large content of vitamins, it is great to keep your red blood cells healthy and guards against oxidative stress. There are some delicious, organic flavors of aloe vera in your local health food store. However, if you are taking diuretics, digoxin or have diabetes, you must avoid consuming too much aloe vera juice because it could lower your blood sugar level. Consult with your doctor.

Kombucha Tea: We feel kombucha tea is such a treasure that we're going to go into detail on this one. Remember, digestion is the key to good health... and there is no better aid to digestion than kombucha tea. You can buy flavored kombucha tea in any health food store, but you'll find it's pretty expensive. We suggest getting in the habit of making it yourself, welcome it into your life, make it part of your family and marry it. We will give you the recipe to make it yourself.

Kombucha is a raw, fermented, probiotic and naturally carbonated tea. You can have it cold or hot, but it is much better cold or room temperature. The hippies of the 1970's embraced home-brewed kombucha tea as a health beverage. However, kombucha tea goes back much further than that. Some records go as far back as the Qin dynasty (220BC). There is evidence that Genghis Khan and his men drank kombucha in the 12th century to stay big and strong with all the pillaging they were doing. Kombucha tea has been popular in Asia, Japan, Korea and Russia.

Kombucha tea is made by mixing water, regular tea, sugar, and a fermenting culture called a SCOBY (Symbiotic Colony of Bacteria and Yeast). It sounds like you might have to be a scientist, but you don't. It's easy. We'll give you a link.

Analysis of the contents of kombucha confirms that it is rich in amino acids, probiotics, antioxidants, glucuronic acid, from Ancient Greek γλυκύς "sweet" is a carboxylic acid), trace minerals, B vitamins and more. It is a living enzyme-rich drink. All of these things are excellent for your digestion and your immune system. Amino acids, glucuronic acid and antioxidants are potentially cancer preventative. So get acquainted.

Herbal Tea with Honey: If everything is going according to plan when you wake up, the right way to keep it going is all natural herbal tea. Typically made hot to give your body the slight nudge into the day it needs, herbal tea is the best practice of keeping the body and mind on even levels.

Hibiscus or green tea, lemongrass, lavender or peppermint ingredients are all good ways to go, and by adding honey for a little sweetness, you'll aid in fighting off sickness and disease. Don't fret over finding and concocting these ingredients together, just buy a good loose-leaf tea that has it done for you already, or just buy quality herbal tea bags. Do yourself a favor and lay off the cheap stuff.A favorite tea beverage is rosehip tea, chamomile, peppermint and 1/3 liquid organic cranberry juice. It looks like wine and tastes great hot or cold. Our girlfriends love this tea with pomegranate juice.

Some people combine herbal teas with juices, like orange juice to make a tea-like smoothie.

ALERT: Toxins, pesticides, soy and GMOs are found in more teas then you could shake a stick at. Please buy organic teas only. There is a great blog about this in www.foodbabe.com

Chai Tea Instead of Coffee: All you really need in the morning is something warm to wake you up. Hot water with lemon will do the trick. Sure, your hands are shaking from caffeine withdrawal, but you can move past that. The best way to wean yourself off caffeine is with a nice hot-spiced chai tea.

The natural ingredients, including ginger root and cloves, provide not only an arguably more interesting flavor than coffee; it's also a healthy and sickness-fighting drink.

If you are dead set on having your coffee, MAKE SURE IT IS ORGANIC. Traditional coffee is incredibly toxic with sprays.

Honey Ginger Lemonade: Ginger-based drinks aid in digestion. Simply add honey and fresh, peeled ginger to fresh squeezed lemon juice and water on top of ice. You can add a little mint to give yourself that "at an expensive resort" feel. Ursula's favorite drink that keeps her strong and healthy is lemon, ginger, and flor-essence tea. Flor- Essence tea is an herbal tea sold as a health tonic with the same herbal components as Essiac tea, a mixture long used in anticancer and AIDS treatments.

Kefir: This is a fermented, beverage, sour mild- high in calcium, potassium and protein. This is one dairy product that we recommend. It offers a wide range of vitamins, mineral and amino acids, and also provides a variety of probiotic organisms and powerful healing qualities. The various types of beneficial microbiota contained in kefir make it one of the most potent probiotic foods available. This beverage has a positive effect on both gut and bone health. Certain bacteria strains from kefir culture have been shown to help in treating colitis by regulating the inflammatory response of the intestinal cells.

Biotta Breuss: This vegetable juice is a blend of fresh organic vegetables such as beet roots, carrots, celery root, potatoes and radishes. It is well suited for juice fasting regimes – but is also delicious as an afternoon treat. This juice has a cleansing and purifying effect on the entire

In addition to all the incredible remedies and recipes that Ursula uses daily, she must say that one product stands out above the rest, Liquid BioCell Life. A delicious nutraceutical supplement filled with fruits, berries, collagen, chondroitin sulfate and hyaluronic acid. This combination is only found together in Liquid BioCell Life and will give your body the most powerful nutrients known today.

Because of the unique liquid delivery system with Mangosteen, Acai Berry, Pomegranate, Blueberry, Lycium, Jujube and more, this formulation has a high antioxidant activity level, which helps create and improve healthy aging, younger looking skin, flexible joints and even helps support healthy cartilage (something we all need as we age). It is also high in phytonutrient antioxidants including Resveratrol. Ursula loves it, and has been consuming Liquid BioCell for the last 4 years. She can say with utmost integrity that she has seen this blend create optimal health for herself and her friends. Experience the benefits of Liquid BioCell Life today. Visit www.liquidcollagensecret.com

body. You can buy Biotta Breuss vegetable juice in many different flavors. Sometimes major chains Costco and Sam's carry it. It is delicious and easy. Please note that since the product is manufactured in Europe, the farms that supply Biotta's raw materials are European Certified Organic. However, due to labeling laws in this country, the bottles sold here cannot state that the product is organic.

For an instant pH shift use one lemon, add 1/4 of pineapple in a blender with 1 cup of coconut water. It's that simple and tastes great! Using lemon and pineapple juice will quickly shift your body pHin your favor! For more information visit Healthwyze.org.

Juicing: We can't say it enough. Vegetable juices are your daily go-to for vitamins and minerals. Juiced carrots, beets, celery and greens will keep young and healthy forever. (Well, maybe not forever, but for a long time)/

You really cannot go wrong. Just try different combinations. Apples and bananas are easy to add to any green drink to give it an extra fruity sweet flavor. Start simple and keep experimenting. Maybe you can go to a juice bar or health food store and try different combinations. There have to be about a zillion recipes online.

Fresh vegetable juices are a great way to increase your base of nutrition. Two of the easiest and most efficient ways to optimize your

Vegetables contain an array of antioxidants and other disease-fighting compounds. Some plant chemicals can reduce inflammation and eliminate carcinogens, while others regulate the rate at which cells reproduce, get rid of old cells and maintain DNA.

vegetable intake is to juice your vegetables and add sprouted seeds such as broccoli seeds, sunflower seeds and pea seeds. There are so many delicious juicing recipes for free on the Internet. You don't have to make it complicated. A very simple start would be carrot and apple! We've provided some very simple recipes.

There has been a long-standing debate as to which style of juice is better, green or mixed vegetables. Carrots provide high levels of beta-carotene, anti-cancerous compounds and alkaline minerals, while green juices are high in chlorophyll, a green pigment that is a natural blood cleanser, and lower in sugar content than carrot juice. The old adage applies "green is clean". The green juices tend to be more bitter than carrot juice, but due to this fact, they are helpful for the liver to purge its bile.

A simple sample green juice: Pat admits that although she had no fewer than three very expensive and complicated juicers at home... able to juice cement if she wanted... her life of serious juicing did not begin until she purchased the Nutri Bullet. This is not an ad for the NutriBullet. We have no stock in them. It is just a simple example of how easy it is to juice when you have the right equipment for the right person.

Her simple green juice recipe that she now drinks 2x per day consists of, basically, what's available fresh and organic at the store. She started out with the organic ingredients simply spinach, green grapes, and protein powder. She has added as time has gone on, and she has changed and experimented constantly with what's fresh and in market. Now she adds celery, cucumbers, moringa leaves from her tree outside, diatomaceous earth, chia seeds, parsley... just name it, she's tried it. Additionally, her husband's organic garden now has six dedicated rows of spinach and kale just for their juicing needs.

Your main goal is to decide which juice to use and begin right now. Juices are an incredible way to boost nutritional levels and ease digestion. They also are one of the best ways to cleanse the blood. You wouldn't stand for dirty gas running your car, right? Get your blood clean and you will be a mean machine!

Wheat grass juice is in a whole category by itself. One ounce of juice is equal to almost two pounds of vegetables. In the nutrition world, it is like putting high octane into your engine. If able, start with one ounce daily and work up to

Sprouts can contain up to 100 times more enzymes than raw fruits and vegetables, allowing your body to extract more vitamins, minerals, amino acids and essential fats from the foods you eat.

The content of vitamins and essential fatty acids increases dramatically during the sprouting process. Depending on the sprout, nutrient content can increase as much as 30 times the original value within just a few days of sprouting and minerals bind to protein during sprouting, making them more bioavailable.

Additionally, the sprouting process deactivates many of the anti-nutrients that are in the seeds.

2 ounces daily. It tastes like your lawn grass and will cause strong detoxification of your body so start with only 1 ounce and gradually work up as tolerated.

Recommendation is 2oz twice a day, it should be noted that the body cannot utilize more than 2oz at a time.

Whether you juice it, or steam it, sauté it, or eat it raw.... All Hail for Kale! This is Ursula's favorite green, and she says, "In Germany we eat Kale in wintertime at least 3x per week. My mother always cooked with what was in season". Just one cup of raw kale will provide 100 percent of your daily needs for vitamins A, C and K. Kale is loaded with antioxidants, calcium and fiber and is available all year. It certainly deserves to be as popular, as or even more popular than spinach or chard. Choose a bunch that is crisp. It comes in green, purple and red winter colors, and you can treat it just like spinach. Keep it wrapped in a damp towel, give it a quick rinse then rip the stems and inner veins from the leaves. The stalks are edible but many people do not like the chewy texture (Ursula saves her stalks for juicing). She also cuts her kale into small pieces and adds it to salad or soups. Kale is delicious sautéed in a pan with a bit of olive oil. Use your imagination. You can also make kale chips by tearing some leafs apart, putting them in a single layer on a baking sheet and drizzling them with olive oil. Sprinkle with salt or other seasonings and you have your new favorite healthy snack.

Kale is a super food but so are these other greens:

- **Bok Choy:** It belongs to the cabbage family, a group known for its anticancer properties probably because of its high concentration of the antioxidant kaempferol.
- **Beet Greens:** They have 60% more potassium than the same amount of spinach. They also contain vitamin A and vitamin K.
- **Chard:** They are loaded with magnesium to hėlp lower blood pressure and can lower the risk of stroke.
- **Mustard Greens:** They may be more effective at lowering cholesterol and decreasing the risk of cardiovascular disease and cancer than cabbage or broccoli.

You agree, right? There is no earthly reason to drink soda, or sugar-filled, corn syrup laden bottled fruit juices. No earthly reason at all. Why in the world would you drink something that would cause you bodily harm when there are so many choices that will aid you in staying healthy, losing weight and feeling great.

Steps to integrate into your daily habits.

- Pay attention to what you really drink each day. You could be enhancing your digestion and your health by making a few simple changes.

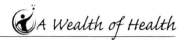

- Have a fresh "green" drink each morning. If you don't like the color green, add beets or carrots to it and change the color. This can actually substitute as your breakfast if you add a little protein powder.
- Drink healthy liquids all thru the day. Mix your Kombucha tea with organic cranberry juice or seltzer water... make it to your liking any healthy way you can.
- Have a pitcher of water always handy with sliced lemons for a refreshing, cleansing drink before each meal.
- Herbal tea is a wonderfully comforting evening snack. You may not be as hungry as you think you are! Have a cup of tea instead.

SELF TEST FOR CHAPTER 4

1. Kombucha tea is...

a. Only available in the Far East
b. Must be sipped while watching cartoons
c. A raw, fermented, probiotics and naturally carbonated tea which is great for digestion; you can make yourself, you can flavor any way you want.

2. You should avoid consuming too much aloe Vera juice if...

a. You live in Florida
b. You are on vacation
c. You are taking diurectics, digoxin or have diabetes (Check with your Doctor)

3. Vegetable juices provide

a. Pretty colors
b. Messy glasses
c. Lots and lots of vitamins and minerals

4. One ounce of wheat grass juice is equal to

a. A small yard in New York City
b. 3 hours of running
c. Almost two pounds of vegetables

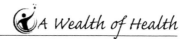

5. It is smart to add sprouts to your juicing because

a. It gives the drink a nice wormy texture
b. You really can't do anything else with sprouts
c. Sprouts can contain up to 100x more enzymes than raw fruits and vegetables.

"Eat right and do what you love. Whatever you love to do is play; doing what you don't like to do is work. I have never worked a day in my life!"

— Dr. Laila Denmark, age 114

Chapter Five

CLEANSING FROM THE INSIDE OUT

You already know that in order to extend the life of your car you need to regularly change the oil and fluid in its radiator. You don't question it you just do it. (We already know you are pretty smart because you bought this book.) Nobody likes to hear this, but every once in a while we need to clean from the inside out. Yes, we're talking about detoxing.

There is only a slight difference between the terms detoxifying and cleansing, and we will use them interchangeably here. Both processes help eliminate toxins from the body, and that's what we're all about. Of course, the primary cause of toxins in our bodies is food additives. However, emotions, the air and our environment, electromagnetic toxicity (i.e. cell phones and computers) and lactic acid content in our muscles are all additional causes of toxicity.

Why cleanse?

Even when we are trying our best, modern times offer some toxic challenges. Eventually, residue from foods with preservatives, chemicals or artificial flavoring which the body cannot assimilate properly, builds up and starts slowing you down. It may even slow you to a stop. Vital organs can just stop functioning properly due to toxic overload. Gallstones, kidney stones, constipation, depression, blood sugar imbalance, insomnia and headaches are some of the beginning symptoms of toxicity. If not addressed, your toxicity can lead to conditions that are even more serious.

Imagine a toxin entering your body. Your immune system will immediately try to push it out through perspiration, saliva, urine, feces, menstruation, earwax, sinuses, the eyes... anywhere it can get it out. If your immune system is unable to keep up with the chore of keeping you clean, it will put the toxins aside wherever it can, until it can get to them later. Your clever body will even, eventually, build little storage tanks for toxins to keep them out of the way while it runs shop.

Picture a lovely little house that keeps getting littered with papers, dust, dirt, plates, clothes, toys - whatever – and you never have the time to really clean it, so you take the debris and shove it under the cushions, the couch, the rug, or in a closet until you have a free Saturday to catch up. Only you never have a free Saturday. Things just keep piling up. Everyday there is more and more litter. Close your eyes briefly and get a clear mental picture before reading on.

In the beginning, this messy house is an irritation to you. When we relate this 'messy house' to the body and toxins – it is the stage of inflammation. That's when the doctor tells you that you have some sort of 'itis'. Arthritis, colitis, dermatitis, tonsillitis... the list goes on and on. "Itis" means inflammation.

Soon, your messy house is becoming hard to navigate. You are tripping over things. So, you build extra closets. You put plastic bins filled with "stuff" in the garage to get it out of the way. Now let's relate this scene to an overwhelmed body that cannot eliminate toxins so it creates little storage tanks for them so that it can get to them later... when there's more time, when it's not so tired, when it hasn't got so much to deal with. Examples of storage tanks that your body builds for toxins are cysts, swellings, cellulite, and benign tumors. This is when the doctor tells you that you have colon polyps, ovarian cysts, fibroid tumors, or obesity.

However, the littering is still going on. So now you have a messy house filled with litter AND storage bins. Are you with me so far?

Here is where the real trouble starts. Imagine that your house is now so filled with litter and storage bins that trash is literally busting through the roof and windows and you have become infested with termites or rats that are eating away at the structure of your home. The beams and framing are being eaten by termites, the electrical wiring is shorting out, and the plumbing is rusting and leaking. Let's relate this to the body. If the body still goes on storing toxins and not cleansing itself, it can lead to cell or DNA damage which leads to the creation of sick, malfunctioning organs, heart attacks, impotence, Crohn's disease, Alzheimer's, Parkinson's and more.

Patricia and Ursula met at a radical detoxification week called the Hawaiian Huna Cleanse. Each day for 7 days they met at someone's home in the woods, drank salt water, meditated, did yoga, spoke with a guru and pooped in a bucket. Then, they lined up with their little filled buckets and presented them to the guru one at a time as he analyzed the contents.

Don't worry. They will not be asking you to do that. Now, anything they say will seem simple to you, right? No worries. You're about to get some tips on how to cleanse a little bit at a time and keep your house clean and tidy on a daily basis. They will also give you the resources to learn about all-out spring-cleaning flushes (which will not be so hard once you are cleansing a little bit each day). It will not be long until you're setting aside weekends to give yourself those extra turbo boosts.

Here's a simple start for daily cleansing:

- Each morning when you wake up have a warm cup of water with fresh lemon juice in it. This simple habit alone will help flush toxins out of your system and give you a nice pick me up in the morning that does not include coffee. Having the water warm is comforting as well as a signal to your body that you are, literally, getting warmed up and ready to go.

As you progress, you won't be happy with just the lemon juice. You will be following that with a shot of Kombucha tea to provide your body with all the probiotics and enzymes it wants, to be running at its best. Then you can have a 'breakfast to go' of fresh juiced spinach, kale and grapes... or any combination of greens and fruits. Voila! You have just managed to provide your body with essential nutrients that will keep you rolling for the next 3 hours at least. One meal down, two to go.

Of course, you do not have to switch to green drinks on a regular basis. If you incorporate the warm lemon water in your daily routine, you will be miles ahead of most people. Not us, but most people.

Now, if you can pick some of the foods from the list below to incorporate into the rest of your meals, you will be continuing the cleansing process all through the day. As if you were roaming around the house dusting this and that all day long.

Cleansing is now down to a science. There are different cleanses with different ingredients for every organ of your body; such as, the kidney cleanse, gallbladder cleanse, liver cleanse, urinary tract cleanse, and intestinal cleanse. Cleansing can help speed the healing of almost every disease. It turns a sluggish body into a vibrant machine.

If you have not already eliminated the following from your diet (and we sincerely hope you have), you will want to do your best to eliminate or minimize them before any major organ or system cleanse. Although I have heard of some people attempting to cleanse while still eating toxic substances, it can make the process uncomfortable for hours or even days. That's because your body's efforts to eliminate will be sabotaged by constant additional toxins causing it to overreact with headaches, stomachaches, joint pain or sheer exhaustion. Do not let this scare you. Imagine trying to clean out your closet while someone keeps throwing clothes in there. Keep in mind that whatever you eliminate or minimize will help your body cleanse that much deeper and faster.

- All coffee (an acidic food that weakens the adrenal function)
- Tobacco
- Alcohol
- All sugar sweet foods and artificial sweeteners (sugar feeds cancer cells and weakens immune function; artificial sweeteners are carcinogenic)

10 top cleansing foods for your body

1. Avocado, high in fiber, potassium, vitamin E and monounsaturated fats
2. Raw coconut cream or coconut oil. Promotes good intestinal environment and has compounds that help remove toxins from body,
3. Flax seeds, chia seeds and hemp seeds or hemp hearts. Fiber, essential fatty acids
4. Raw cultured sauerkraut or veggies – have billions of live probiotics
5. Blueberries high in fiber, low in sugar, powerful antioxidants – super food
6. Resveratrol – a phytonutrient found in grapes said to reverse the effects of aging and fight cancer
7. Cucumbers, minerals, fiber and hydrating ability
8. Tomatoes fiber high Vitamin C and antioxidant lycopene,
9. Raw milk kefir, yogurt billions of friendly microbes and support healthy digestion
10. Kombucha... try it with chia seeds

If you added one or more of the above foods to your diet each day, you would be helping your body eliminate toxins on a continuous basis. This is the easiest way to vibrant health. What you do day after day has the largest impact on your body. It would also make it much easier to do some "spring cleaning" or a major system cleanse, because it would not be as drastic.

- All fried food and fatty foods as fats feed tumors
- All white flour products (converts to sugar & is mucus forming)
- All cow based dairy products i.e. milk, cheese, ice cream, etc. (mucus forming which compounds cancer cell activity)
- All refined processed foods (As Jack LaLane used to say, "If man made it don't eat it!")
- Reduce or avoid all meats, especially any preserved meats. (Any meat is acidic; however, the nitrates in preserved meats such as hot dogs and cold cuts are highly carcinogenic.)
- All soda products
- All added salt products. If using any salt on food use only very sparingly and add only sea salt.
- All forms of milk chocolate should be avoided.
- Partially hydrogenated oils

What this means is that you MUST be consuming fresh natural foods in their whole form! If the food is refined in any way, it is devoid of its essential nutrients and altered with chemicals, which becomes harmful and weakening to the body. There is no sense in trying to swim upstream. You're not a salmon.

Dr. Schulze at www.herbdoc.com has some good teas and herbal formulas to help you cleanse all the nonsense away. So does www.blessedherbs.com Another great source for cleanses is Dr. Robert Morse, author of *The Detox Miracle Sourcebook*, www.drmorsesherbalhealth club.com

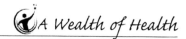

We would like to suggest that every so often you take a few days and have nothing but fresh-juiced greens. Don't worry, you won't die. You'll probably lose a few pounds and feel like a new person. Some of our friends might find the time to do this once a year. Others set aside a weekend every month or two. You can tell by looking into their eyes which is which.

Another route to take is The Master Cleanse Recipe. It works just like it sounds. You consume primarily lemonade for the entire time you are on this regime. Therefore, the recipes for the diet itself are fairly simple. You should drink a minimum of 60 oz of lemonade a day, but can drink more if you like. You can also drink as much water as you want.

Below is a recipe for 60 ounces of the Master Cleanse, which will get you through one glorious day.

- 60 ounces of filtered water
- 12 tablespoons of organic Grade B maple syrup
- 12 tablespoons of organic lemon juice
- ½ teaspoon cayenne pepper powder

There are a couple of important things to remember when preparing the lemonade. The lemon juice used must be fresh squeezed. This cannot be emphasized enough. It is necessary to use fresh produce. Canned juice will not work and will erase most of the benefits of using the master cleanse diet.

In addition, the maple syrup must be organic grade B maple syrup, not the sugar filled syrup that is used at the typical breakfast table.

The cayenne pepper might seem unnecessary, but it is actually very important. Not only does it help to add a bit of a kick, but also the pepper helps to break up mucus and increases healthy blood flow. It also is a good source of B and C vitamins, commonly referred to as Super Vitamins due to their many benefits for the body.

Learn more at www.themastercleanse.com

Another excellent book on cleansing is: *Cleansing or Surgery by Embassy of Heaven*. www.cleansingorsurgery.com

For some great cleansing juicing recipes, go to www.greenjuiceaday.com or www.thejuicenut.com

Patricia likes using the 10-Day Transformation Cleanse by Purium that meets all of her criteria of soy-free, dairy-free, GMO-free and certified organic. It's simple, yet effective to give you a jump start on helping you realize what your body would feel like toxin-free. Go to www.mypurim.com/healthandbeauty

YOUR LYMPHATIC SYSTEM – A TEAM OF HOUSE MAIDS

Pat and Ursula have saved the explanation of your lymphatic system until now because it is responsible for removing the toxins and waste cell by cell into your elimination system. Imagine a team of maids walking from room to room in your home picking up every piece of litter and debris and bringing it to the outside trash. Dusting and polishing all day long. It is a beautiful system and it would be in our best interests to make sure we keep those maids working smoothly. There are things you can do to help keep your lymphatic system moving freely.

You will want to make sure those maids are free to do their jobs before you start emptying closets and bins, right? Unlike the circulatory system, which is driven by our huge power pump, (the heart), the lymphatic system has no power of its own. All the pathways of the lymphatic system run alongside the circulatory system. When your circulation is pumping, it stimulates the lymphatic system to pump alongside it. This is one reason why exercise is so very important. One of the best all around exercises to stimulate your lymphatic system is rebounding. To save your knees, use a small trampoline. However, walking, walking, walking and more walking makes your lymphatic system sing.

Proper hydration is of the utmost importance to this system. And, since you've already committed to hydrating in our digestion section, we are good to go here. So, that leaves skin brushing.

Lymphatic System Boosters

- Proper Hydration
- Exercise and body Movement
- Skin Brushing
- Rebounding (Bouncing up and down on a trampoline

Easy as pie and it feels good, too! Get yourself a nice skin brush (boar bristle is best, but use what you can get and start brushing!). Always remember to brush in the direction of your heart. Up the legs, toward your heart, up the arms, toward your heart, in a clockwise circle around your abdomen. You can go any direction you like on the back (if you can reach it).

A great book on the lymphatic system and skin brushing is *Vital Chi Skin-Brushing System* by Bruce Berkowsky, N.M.D.

OK. Now you're ready for the big time! If you feel you have been cleansing daily for a while and you have your toxins down to a tame few and your lymphatic system operating at full speed, you'll want to bring out the big guns and carefully cleanse one organ system at a time. You can find many wonderful cleansing protocols on the internet for each system of your body. When cleansing system by system it is important to follow a logical order. If you detox your blood with a clogged liver, where do the toxins go? If you detox your liver with a toxic colon, your liver will just get clogged again. Therefore, first you will detoxify your Large Intestine (colon), and work on the kidneys simultaneously. Next, you will detox your liver and gallbladder. Lastly, you will detox your blood. When the liver and blood are detoxified, circulation is improved.

Here's the proper order for individual organ system cleanses.

- Large Intestine (colon)/Kidneys
- Liver/Gallbladder
- Blood

So remember always that in cleansing, start with the bowels or colon. The age-old saying, "all disease starts in the intestine" is a good reminder to start with the intestines. Naturally, in order to keep your bowels beautiful you must be eating plenty of fiber. See Chapter 4.

There are also easy coffee enemas or cocktail enemas to do, but they work on the large intestines and the liver simultaneously. Therefore, we have saved them for later to be sure you do some simple initial cleanses first before partaking of your first coffee enema.

In order to cleanse the colon, along with any other organ, you must change your diet. Diet is key in this process because regardless of the supplements, tools and treatments, you must begin to eat natural foods with the proper nutrients. Eat the foods that treat constipation. The necessary foods are foods that are high in soluble fiber, which is naturally hydrated, and this helps lubricate the intestinal wall and makes it easier for elimination.

In addition, consider using an herbal colon cleanse product of choice. There are various forms on the market, many containing the same base ingredients.

Bitter foods are better for the liver... and also help with colon cleansing. Simply tasting bitter foods on your tongue stimulates bile flow from the liver, which plays an important role in stimulating peristalsis in the intestine. Peristalsis is the wave like muscular activity that moves our waste through our intestine. Adding bitter foods in the diet not only helps cleanse the liver, but also the intestine. (This is why the coffee enema is so effective.) Human beings all throughout the planet originally included bitter foods in their diet, and throughout the years have replaced this key component with sweet and salty foods due to the amount of industrialized processed foods consumed. Proper hydration lubricates the intestinal walls, which aids the elimination of waste.

As far as supplemental herbs available to help with a good colon cleanse, a good standing product is Dr. Shultz Intestinal 2 formula. Blessed Herbs also provides individual cleansing programs for the bowels.

KIDNEYS

You can simultaneously cleanse the kidneys while cleansing the colon.

Easy steps for kidney cleanse:

- Cut a bunch of parsley into smaller pieces.
- Boil the parsley in a pot of water for 10 minutes.
- Let it cool down and then sieve and discard the parsley.

- Pour the filtered water into bottles or any container and keep in fridge.
- Drink one glass of the water daily.
- You should notice the sediments in your urine.

- You should feel a sense of well-being after that.

Some simpler kidney flush ideas:

- Drink watermelon juice (if available) throughout the day.

- Make your own Kidney Flush Tea. Use one bag of a kidney tea (there are many variations). A good tea for the kidneys will often contain juniper berries, gravel root, hydrangea, corn silk, uva ursi, marshmallow root, dandelion root, pipsesewa.

- Alternatively, use about 4-6 ounces of any of the above dry herbs and place into 96 ounces of apple juice, the juice of 10 lemons or limes, 10 ounces of raw apple cider vinegar. Let this mixture stand on your counter over night. The next day strain and drink 4 ounces on the hour every hour for two days.

Now that the bowels are open, it is a perfect time to flush the liver! Over time, the environment, poor diet and lifestyle choices, especially alcohol consumption, acetaminophen, non-prescription painkillers, and all the toxins and garbage in our used-to-be regular diet, (Think sodas, candy, GMOs), adversely affect the liver.

The liver is actually the largest solid organ in our bodies, and it works extremely hard. As discussed in Chapter 2, the liver has over 500 different functions. One of its most important functions is to filter the blood that comes from the digestive tract and get all those toxins out of the body. Do you understand why you want to eat as cleanly as possible? The liver also converts waste products from metabolic functions into urea to be eliminated by urine. It creates bile to help digest fats and carbohydrates. Besides balancing blood sugars and creating red blood cells, it also synthesizes glutathione, the master antioxidant that also helps recycle other spent antioxidants.

A basic cheap liver flush:

First thing in the morning:

- One clove garlic
- One tablespoon olive oil
- 8 ounces citrus juice
- Quarter cup fresh parsley

Blend and drink. To strengthen, increase the garlic by one clove or the olive oil by one tablespoon to suit your tolerance. Five would be the max. Wait a half hour to an hour and drink 2 cups of a detox tea as a chaser.

An easy liver cleanser:

First thing in the morning:

8-10 apricots in the blender with water. Drink the fluid and then eat the pits. This stimulates the bile flow, lubricates and hydrates the intestine.

A stronger liver flush:

Step 1 Prep for 3 days: 32 ounces of apple juice or citrus juice (8 lemons) to pre-soften bile and gallstones

Step 2 On the 3rd day: half teaspoon of Epsom salts in four ounces of water exactly at 6pm. (Epsom salts are Magnesium, which dilates the common bile duct and allows for stone and bile to flow.)

Step 3 Repeat at 8pm

Step 4 10pm take one cup of olive oil, the juice of one grapefruit shake and drink quickly.

Step 5 Immediately lie in bed, curl your legs up in fetal position. If nauseous chew on a little bit of ginger to settle the stomach.

Step 6 On the following morning at 8am take Epsom salts and water

Step 7 10am repeat step 6. Compliment this Step 7 with a couple of cups of detox tea.

Look for small stones the size of peas or golf balls congealed in olive oil. Another thing to compliment liver cleansing is hot castor oil packs over the liver to help open the liver and flush.

Coffee Enemas and Cocktail Enemas

Because coffee enemas cleanse the liver as well as the colon, we suggest that you do these after you have already cleansed your colon and lymphatic system. Fifteen years ago, Ursula saw a movie during her cancer treatment in Mexico that recommended doing a coffee enema on a daily basis. As first she was hesitant but then they showed everyone a movie of how it works. Ursula has been doing it ever since.

They showed everyone that if you drink coffee, it is acid to the body, but if you do it as an enema it alkalizes the body. It goes into your blood system and stimulates all your organs. At times, Ursula added Flor-essence tea along with probiotics (open up the probiotics capsule and add it to the coffee or tea). If you want to use a probiotic, make sure it has at least 30 billion active microorganisms per capsule.

Here are 10 Reasons Why You Should Try a Coffee Enema:

1. Reduces levels of toxicity by up to 600%.
2. Cleans and heals the colon, improving peristalsis.
3. Increases energy levels, improves mental clarity and mood.
4. Helps with depression, bad moods, and sluggishness.
5. Helps eliminate parasites and Candida.
6. Improves digestion, bile flow, eases bloating.
7. Detoxifies the liver and helps repair the liver.
8. Can help heal chronic health conditions (along with following a mainly raw plant based diet).

9. Helps ease "die-off" or detox reactions during periods of fasting or juice fasting, cleansing or healing.
10. Used regularly in the Gerson Institute treatment protocol for healing Cancer patients naturally.

A lifetime of living on a so-called normal diet can block the liver. As you start to eat and drink the nutrient rich foods, the cells are rapidly absorbing and forcing toxins from the cells into the bloodstream, which in turn transports them to the liver, the body's chief organ of detoxification. As a result the liver may be unable to deal with the newly arriving toxins driven from the tissues by live nutrients. Unless quickly shifted, this logjam of toxins could lead to threatening self-intoxication and liver coma, hence the vital role of rapidly detoxifying with coffee enemas.

It is vital to remove the dead toxic material from the liver. Three scientists from the Department of Pathology, University of Minnesota, confirmed Dr. Max Gerson's use of coffee enemas to detoxify the liver. The tests proved that rectal coffee administration stimulates an enzyme system in the liver, which is able to remove toxic free radicals from the bloodstream. The normal activity of this enzyme is increased by 600-700% by the coffee enemas. This greatly increases detoxification, is rich in potassium, and helps prevent intestinal cramping. A recent 1990 study of six years with a group of 60 cancer patients had amazing results, including reduction in all pain medications, slowing liver metastases, and even complete remission without conventional therapy.

Coffee Enema Instructions

For one Coffee Enema:

- 3 large rounded tablespoons of organic ground coffee in 2 cups boiling water. Bring to slow boil, remove from heat and let stand 15 minutes. Drain coffee grounds and you are left with a coffee concentrate.
- Place coffee concentrate in the enema bucket or enema bag and fill with distilled water to equal a total of 32 ounces. Lie on your right side and slowly add coffee into rectum. If an urge to expel occurs, stop and wait until urge diminishes. Continue filling colon. If you must expel, stop, expel and then continue filling with remaining coffee liquid. Lay in fetal position for 15 min on right side. After 5 minutes, slowly sit up and expel.

Cilantro is a wonderful herb for helping to cleanse heavy metals out of the body. How do heavy metals get in the body? No, not by rocking out. Usually it's due to fillings from the dentist.

Even if you're sensitive to caffeine, it won't affect you taking your coffee this way. (Definitely do not attempt to use decaf coffee though, you won't get the benefits.)

Detox Teas are very helpful and aid the liver, kidneys, lymph and colon. It is helpful to alternate your teas every month or two. The longer amount of time we consistently eat the same foods or herbs, the more the body becomes sensitized by them. Historically we had changes of season, which forced us to alter our diets. Now we have the "convenience" of having the same food sources available to use each day.

Well established detox teas:

- Essiac tea 4-8 ounces daily
- Jason Winter's tea 8-32 ounces daily
- Dr. Schultz detox tea 32 ounces daily
- Huilda Clark's herbal detox tea

When making the teas be sure to use pure water, and make in glass or stainless steel pots. Boil as directed and steep overnight before straining. The longer steeping times will help to increase the potency of the teas.

Two Day Cell Cleanse This Cellular cleanse is one more delicious body cleaning tool. You can do this for 2 days every other month.

12 oranges

6 lemons

6 grapefruit

On Day One, drink this all day long with water. On Day Two take some organic, peeled potatoes and boil them. Take the broth and drink it. It is filled with potassium. In the evening, have as much carrot juice as you would like.

Sweat therapy or hyperthermia is also a long-standing therapy dating back to Hippocrates. The systemic heat induction opens the circulation, moves the lymph, and the sweating helps the body eliminate waste. Every degree of temperature increase in the body doubles the speed activity of your white blood cells. In addition, cancer cells have demonstrated an inability to tolerate temperatures above 101 degrees.

Steam saunas, far-infrared saunas, zone steam saunas are all great ways to help eliminate waste, increase immune response, and provide a hostile environment for cancer cells.

On a sunny summer day, one can often just roll up the windows of the car and park directly into the sun and in just a few minutes have a sauna. Hint: Do not fall asleep.

Hot Epsom salt and baking soda baths are also a good way to compliment hyperthermia. Just take 2-4 cups of Epsom salts and 1 cup of baking soda. Epsom salts are all magnesium and sodium, which makes an isotonic solution that helps to draw waste from the body. Baking soda is an alkaline neutralizer and has even been demonstrated to be helpful in reducing radiation's harmful effects on the body. (Take this bath after airline flights!)

It is best to have a water filtration system in place before using the hot bath therapies as common municipal water sources are high in chlorine and a wide range of harmful chemicals. You can absorb a pound of water weight within one hour of soaking in water, so be sure the water is clean before pursuing bath therapies. If using the bath therapies, be sure to get the water as hot as tolerated and soak at least 30 minutes.

Another easy form of hydrotherapy that should be included in your health routine is hot and cold showers. Be sure to have a shower filter on your shower to reduce the amounts of harmful chemicals. Alternate the water temperature as hot as you can tolerate for 2-3 minutes and then turn the hot water off and use cold water for 2-3 minutes alternate back and forth as long as tolerated each day to help move lymph flow. Hand held shower attachments are great to use since they allow focusing directly to areas of concern. The hot water increases the circulation and the cold water restricts the circulation, giving a forceful pumping movement to your lymphatics.

Often, after you begin eating more cleansing foods and participating in some major tissue and organ cleanses, you realize that you have been operating on 60% capacity for years. Just because you don't FEEL toxic right now, doesn't mean you aren't. Wait. You'll see.

Steps to Integrate into your life to cleanse

- Each morning have a warm water with lemon before anything else.

(this is so important... see how it keeps getting mentioned?)

- Get used to Kombucha tea and start drinking it regularly
- Stop putting toxins IN.
  Check your ingredients

- Try juicing for just one day each week.
- Try having a weekend of just juices.
- It helps to have a friend do this with you

Self Test for Chapter Five

1. The primary causes of toxins in our body are

a. Chemicals and preservatives in food
b. Chemicals in our air and environment
c. Electromagnetic
d. All of the above

2. When toxins build up in our body they can cause

a. Anything ending in 'itis'
b. Degenerative diseases
c. Cellulite and weight gain
d. All of the above

3. We can keep our body on the road to cleansing each day with

a. Warm water and lemon
b. Kombucha tea
c. Green drinks
d. All of the above

4. Before we begin a cleansing program we need to

a. Make sure our lymphatics are working smoothly

b. Put a hold on the mail

c. Shut off our cell phones.

5. The proper order to begin cleansing is

a. Lymphatics, Large Intestine/Kidney, Liver/ Gallbladder

b. Large Intestine, Liver, Kidney, Lymphatics, Gallbladder

c. Kidney, Gallbladder, Liver, Large Intestine, Lymphatics

"Just Live, Love and Laugh
if you want to get along."
Anne Acerra, age 93 (Patricia's Mom!)

Chapter Six

MINDFULNESS – THE ENERGETIC BODY

What does Mindfulness have to do with Digestion?

You cannot separate your physical health from your mental, emotional or spiritual health. They all tie into each other constantly. Practicing happy mood-lifting habits is like strengthening your savings account for a healthy body.

Remember we told you that your stomach was considered your second brain? That's because your body contains a separate nervous system in your gut that is so complex it has been dubbed the second brain. It comprises about 500 million neurons and stretches from your esophagus to your anus. This mass of neural tissue does much more than just handle our digestion. This brain could be responsible for seeking out comfort foods during times of stress, of craving chips and chocolate, and of moods and behavior, and of course, controlling digestion. Your second brain can either work alone – or in conjunction with the brain in your head and may determine mental states as well as play a role in diseases throughout the body.

In Chinese medicine, theories developed over 3,000 years ago attributed over thinking and worry as one of the major reasons for damaging the stomach meridian. The nerves in our gut probably influence big parts of our emotions. Butterflies in the stomach are a physiological signal of stress. Everyday emotional well-being may rely on messages from our second brain to our "head" brain. Studies are now being done linking the serotonin in our enteric nervous system to diseases such as osteoporosis and autism. In fact, the field of 'neurogastroenterology' is growing and will likely shed light on many links between the body and the mind.

The gastrointestinal tract is sensitive to emotion. Every emotion can trigger symptoms in the gut, from butterflies, to nausea. Just the thought of eating can release stomach's juices before the food even gets there. This connection goes both ways! A person's intestinal distress can be either the cause or the result of anxiety, stress or depression. The second brain (your gut) and the 'head' brain are so intimately connected that we should really view them as one system.

In addition, at least 70% of our immune system is in our 'gut', ready to protect us from foreign invaders. Knowing this, you can easily see how stress and negative thinking can weaken your immune system. So think twice, with BOTH your brains, to keep yourself healthy. Pick out one or more practices that relieve stress and help develop mindfulness. Raise your vibrational energy level in a good way.

"Everything is energy and that's all there is to it. Match the frequency of the reality you want and you cannot help but get that reality . It can be no other way. This is not philosophy. This is physics."

-Albert Einstein

ENERGY

Energy, frequency and vibration are the secrets of the universe. People who follow a metaphysical path for higher spirituality have a phrase they use "vibrating at a higher frequency." Watch the video on the web site below at your earliest convenience to see exactly what happens in the physical world when we vibrate at a higher frequency. The video is of an experiment using sand on a metal plate. The sand forms ever more intricate and beautiful patterns as the frequency is raised higher and higher. It is beautiful and amazing. By the way, the "hertz" which is the measurement of frequency is the German word for "heart". http://io9.com/the-most-incredible-thing-youll-watch-today-is-this-video-511739457

We are electromagnetic beings. Each nerve and pulse in our body is an electric current. Every cell we have acts like a tiny battery feeding chemical energy power to our muscles, nerves, organs, and every fiber of our being.

The definition of vibrational frequency is "the rate at which the atoms and sub-particles of a being or an object vibrate. The higher this vibration frequency is, the closer it is to the frequency of light source.

Every thought, every word, every feeling has its own vibrational frequency... its own electrical current. Some of these frequencies are incredibly healing to our body, and some of them are destructive. Each word we speak and every thought we think sends out a vibration that attracts a similar experience. If we send out anger, we attract anger. If we send out love, we attract love.

Every person vibrates at their own unique frequency, which is a mixture of everything they have ever experienced. Those frequencies that we focus our attention on, increase within us. If we focus on doubt, fear, hatred, anger, jealousy, envy, judgment (of either ourselves or others)... we are focusing on lower vibrations. If we focus on love, harmony, peace, balance, kindness, understanding, compassion, etc., we are focusing on higher vibrations. This is one reason that positive affirmations, practiced on a continuous basis throughout the day, can bring such positive results.

HELPFUL HINT: If negative people surround you, look deeply within yourself. We attract people of the same vibrational frequency as ourselves.

Every cell has its own distinct energetic pattern. Each organ, every energy meridian, each chakra, every emotion, all possess their own energetic frequency that can either be nourished or destroyed. Therefore, on a continuous basis, through every word and feeling, we are either raising our energy or lowering it.

Most people think they're doing just fine; they have it all covered. They don't feel stressed - just busy that's all. However, stress is like a drone hovering over you blocking out the sun. Naturally, we cannot avoid all stress, or make it all go away. Yet, we can feed ourselves with positive energy from other sources to protect ourselves from the negative effects of it.

Take some time just for you. Feed yourself with positive frequencies and uplifting energy. Not only will this afford a protection for your body from all the negative frequencies and vibrations that we are still subjected to, but also your body will respond with a bounce in your step... a lilt in your voice... an aura of peace and happiness and health all around you. Your cup runneth over. You'll be spilling an energetic elixir all over anyone you meet. You'll look better!

In ancient wisdom, our physical body extends outward in seven layers penetrating the previous ones, and all disease and dysfunction begins when our extended bodies take on negative vibrations. Quantum physicists have proven that we are not just our physical bodies. Our presence extends beyond our skin line. We have an energy field around us. Kirlian photography has proven this. Our health, our consciousness and our thoughts can all change our energy field.

Refer to the book "Messages From Water" by Dr. Masoru Emoto to see how words can actually change the molecular structure of water (remember, our bodies are over 60% water!) Here is a video that shows it in action: www.youtube.com/watch?v=L0JU03CGFrUIf considering your physical health from the aspect of spiritual and emotional health just does not resonate with you, look to the body of scientific evidence being accumulated day after day, which shows how stress can weaken your immune system, cause disease, and wear you down. Stress is just another word for negative vibrations... or anything that you wish were different.

"We have a thinking immune system that eavesdrops on our thoughts."
- Deepak Chopra, M.D.

Any stress in our life robs us of energy. Take deep breaths of fresh air. Stand with your face to the sun. Put your bare feet on the earth, or on a shoreline. Listen to the sound of moving water. Meditate, pray, love. Take care of your mental, emotional and spiritual self in whatever way resonates with you. Make lists of everything that stirs you in a good way... whether it's the sound of a child's laughter, hugging a dog, watching a sunset, and then make sure you give yourself opportunities to enjoy those things! This is not selfish. This is healthy living. Allow yourself those things that nourish you.

The easiest way, of course, to be sure that our mental, emotional and spiritual state supports good health is to be on an ascended path. This means to feel our connection with a Higher Power and love and peace and oneness, and never get caught in the negative swirls of this earthly life. Pursuing spiritual growth, compassion in daily life, connection to others, forgiveness of yourself and others, are all ways of someone on the ascended path. These are all ways to raise our vibrational frequency.

However, we are human and it is hard to come from spirit all the time when you are living in a material world. Therefore, we are going to share some mindfulness practices with you that help keep many people calm, happy, and healthy on a continuous basis. We hope you try some out and that they feed you with positive vibrations.

Stand on the Earth: Let's start from the ground up. Literally. Walk barefoot in the grass, on the sand or on the soil. Walking on concrete is OK, as is walking barefoot on tiles in your home. Gardening is also very good. How simple is THAT? Scientific evidence is showing that this practice, called "Earthing" works wonders for your body. Earthing makes the blood flow better. Your body instantly absorbs electrons from the earth, which help to diminish inflammation in the body. It is calming. Earthing works because the earth resonates at 7.83 Hz and when we connect to it, the earth will calm and heal our bodies. Standing barefoot in the sand by the ocean also works, and don't underestimate the power of hugging a tree.

Traditional health care systems like Chinese and Ayurvedic medicine have promoted the health benefits of skin contact with the earth for hundreds, if not thousands of years. Now, recent research into the effects of earthing is showing that it leads to an increase in parasympathetic nervous system activity, and reduces sympathetic activity. Anything that promotes parasympathetic activity is sorely needed in this day and age as we are constantly in a state of sympathetic hyperdrive. Earthing is being proven to normalize cortisol secretion (the reason behind abdominal fat) and normalize melatonin secretion (which will aid in better sleep). Earthing also has a powerful anti-inflammatory affect by absorbing electrons from the earth to fight free radicals. For more scientific information go to www.earthinginstitute.net

Water: If you live anywhere near a body of water... whether it is an ocean, gulf, river, stream, creek or lake, go visit it. Just watching water flow soothes the mind and emotions. Close your eyes and listen to it splash. Healing, right? Stick your feet in it. Jump in it. Play in it. Water is the most nurturing of all the elements. Honor it. Bring a consciousness to your bath or shower and imagine all your mental, emotional or spiritual toxins just sliding down the drain.

Meditate: Oh, I can hear the groans from here. But listen, it's not that hard. Don't fall for that concept that you have to erase every single thought from your head; it is not going to happen. At least not at first. Let the thoughts pass through you and soon there will be fewer and fewer. Meditation is something you can practice anywhere, anytime (except while you're driving). Meditation is simply a relaxed state of being and there are many techniques to get you there. For simple starters, use the mantra meditation technique and repeat a phrase over and over to yourself until you sort of self-hypnotize. Try this one: "I am one with source." If that's too weird for you right now, then just say, "I am at peace." Say whatever you want – as long as it's positive.

Hypnotherapy: Hypnotherapy is a state of deep relaxation where you can set aside the critical factor in your conscious mind and access your sub- conscious mind. Your subconscious mind is the seat of your emotions and habits and belief systems – and really runs the show. It's the "Man behind the curtain", so to speak. In an hypnotic state you can give your subconscious mind new directives to work with you to achieve your goals of health and happiness, clear away old dysfunctional belief systems that have held you back from peace and prosperity, release and heal traumatic memories, and bring yourself to a solid core state of happiness. Whether you use tapes, guided meditations, or see a hypnotherapist for specific and deep work, you will be amazed at the calming feeling of inner power and wholeness you can experience, and how empowered you become to make the changes you need. For free Monday night classes explaining principles of your mind and healing, (along with incredible guided meditations) go to www.tfioh.com

Tai Chi or Qi Gong are two more mind body practices that originated in China. Let's face it, when it comes to stress reduction our Eastern brothers and sisters are way ahead of us. These gentle and beautiful flowing movements evolved, believe it not, from martial arts. Think of a moving meditation. You can work individually with a teacher, take a class, or buy a video. It's fun, it's challenging in a good way, and you can do this whether you're 5 or 105. If you need something the whole family can do, Tai Chi or Qi Gong might be the ticket.

Prayer: That's right. Numerous scientific studies have shown that regular prayer is an important factor in living longer and staying happy and healthy. Over 85% of people confronting a major illness pray. Why does it take a crisis to bring us to our knees? There's a relaxation response which occurs in prayer according to studies done at Harvard Medical School. If you are someone who has been praying since childhood, then you already know this. If you're someone who has never tried it, you may be pleasantly surprised at the peace of mind and calmness that ensues. No direction needed. Just go off by yourself and say what is in your heart – or don't say anything at all. Just envision a beam of light from your heart to the heavens. It works. Simply focusing in on your heart and feeling gratitude for whatever it is you have is one of the most powerful prayers there is.

Acupuncture: Acupuncture is one of the key components of traditional Chinese medicine and is among the oldest energetic healing practices in the world. Recent scientific studies have proven the existence of pathways and points on the body that were recorded thousands of years ago. Specific points are stimulated to unblock any blockages of energy (or Qi) whether the cause is mental, emotional, or physical. This helps the body gently return to a state of well-being, health and mental clarity. Esoteric acupuncture specifically helps to clear chakras and your human energy field (aura) which has seven levels. These levels are often referred to as subtle energy bodies and each one has a different vibrational frequency.

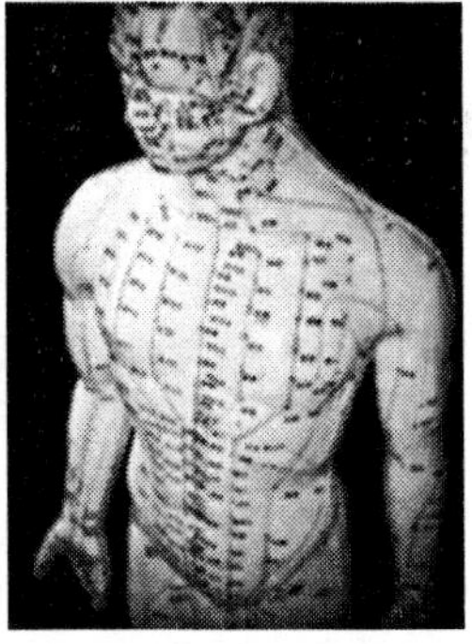

Yoga: The word "yoga" comes from the Sanskrit root "yuj" which means "to yoke" the spirit and physical body together. Yoga has evolved over thousands of years to embrace a wide range of styles and disciplines. Yoga is a popular activity for athletes, children, and seniors. Yoga can be modified to suit all levels of fitness. Yoga has been proven to lower blood pressure and increases strength and flexibility. Yoga energizes our bodies and calms our minds.

Massage: Massage is one of the most relaxing, comforting, preventative modalities out there. Where else can you just lie there and do nothing, feel really good, and simultaneously be strengthening your immune system, enhancing your circulation, helping your respiratory system, nervous system and organs of elimination, and toning your muscles at the same time. Yes, massage does all that. It is not self-indulgence. It's one of the most enjoyable methods of preventative medicine that anyone could ever use. Next birthday, ask for a gift certificate.

Chakra Healing: In Hindu and Buddhism metaphysical tradition as well as other belief systems, chakras are centers of life force or vital energy. They are vortexes of energy at specific points along the center line of our body, each vortex dealing with a different aspect of our life and the emotions associated with that aspect. One result of an energetic imbalance among your chakras (such as a blocked chakra) is an almost continuous feeling of dissatisfaction. Other dysfunctions can include, looking outside for fulfillment, anxiety, or a loss of touch with your true feelings.

There are many ways to balance your chakras and once you start researching it, you are sure to find something simple you'd like to try. Almost every energy modality, including Reiki, Yoga, Emotional Freedom Technique, Breathwork, Acupuncture, Aromatherapy, Meditation, and more, addresses healing your chakras. Now that you have had this brief explanation, we hope you experiment. The results are a calming, centered and grounded feeling of well-being.

These Cause Acidity in your Body		
Anger	**Tension**	**Worry**
Fear	**Jealousy**	**Resentment**
Hate	**Overwork**	**Lack of sleep**
	Stress	

A beautiful little book you may want to buy for yourself is "The Four Agreements" by Don Miguel Ruiz. He covers the following directives coupled with meditations:

1. Be impeccable with your word
2. Don't take anything personally
3. Don't make assumptions
4. Always do your best

The Silva Method: This is a therapeutic technique sometimes grouped under the name human potential movement. Ursula went to the seminar 25 years ago and says, "I thought it was very 'out there'. I have a different point of view on it now and still use the method to this day. Each day I meditate between 5-20 minutes."

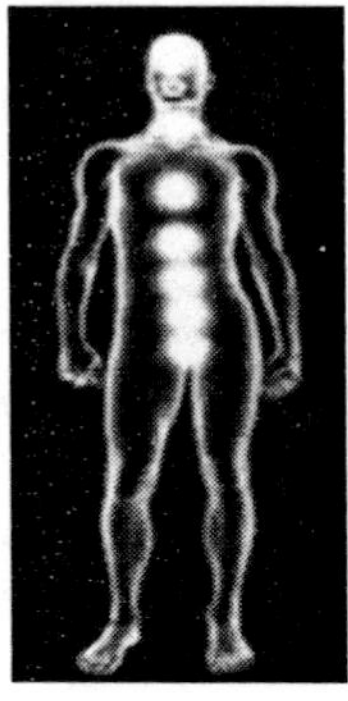

You create a happy place in your mind that brings back good memories. Ursula's happy place is a sailboat on the ocean. Pat's happy place is deep in a forest. You breathe in and breathe out 10 breaths, counting backward from 10 to one. If you count, your brain will be clear. Imagine yourself in the happy place and bring awareness to the surrounding there such as, sight, smell, sound and touch. You get lost in space because you are so immersed in this positive experience. When you are ready, take a deep breath and release yourself from the happy place and you should feel refreshed.

Emotional Freedom Technique: This modality is based on the subtle energy system of acupuncture meridians. It is a new Western application of these 5,000-year-old principles. Energy is transported through our body via acupuncture meridians. If the energy flow is disrupted, we can experience unease, pain, discomfort. With physical tapping at specific points along our energy meridians, we can keep it balanced and running smoothly. www.healing-with-eft.com!

Seven Day Mental Diet: Ursula read this book 30 years ago and has continued to refer to it periodically. Basically, you commit yourself to saying ONLY positive statements for seven full days. If you mess up, you have to start over. That's seven full days without holding or expressing a negative thought for more than 60 seconds. It sounds easy. Try it. The download for the seven day mental diet is http://vst.-cape.com/~rch/fox.html

Ursula loves the workshops from Donna Eden and still does her 5 minutes Energy routine before getting out of bed.
http://www.youtube.com/watch?v=gffKhttrRw4
This is the link to the teaching of Donna Eden's 5 Minute Energy Routine

Seven Day Mental Diet:
Habits of Happy People

- Be kind to everyone
- Have big dreams
- Don't make excuses
- Live in the now
- Express gratitude
- Let problems stimulate your intellect
- Don't compare yourself to others
- Speak well of everyone
- Speak well of yourself
- Stay in touch with your friends
- Meditate daily-pray
- Be honest
- Listen instead of talking
- Minimize TV time
- Get out in Nature
- Keep moving
- Get a little sun each day
- Know what you like and pursue it
- Make lists - goals
- Create, paint, cook, garden
- Repeat affirmations
- Laugh, laugh, laugh
- Love, love, love
- Sing and smile
- Always do your best
- Don't assume anything
- Don't take anything personally

Roger Callahan, PhD, authored several best-selling books about accessing our energy system within. Among those books are *Tapping The Healer Within, Tapping the Body's Energy Pathways; Tapping Nature's Healing System,* and *Thought Field Therapy Boot Camp*. Thought Field Therapy is a process combining principles of Western and Eastern healing methods, using energy points in the body to release emotional distress. His protocols have helped thousands of people eliminate fears and phobias, calm stress, and reveal and heal what is holding them back from success. You can get the books or CDs from www.rogercallahan.com

Also, go on *YouTube* for tapping tips.

Biofeedback: This is a viable modality used in the energetic identification and correction of mind/body stressors. It stimulates the body's own self-healing mechanisms with the possibility of preventing and alleviating disease and disorders. Since 4,000 B.C., healers have understood that our health greatly depends on the quality of energy that flows through and makes up our bodies. The latest scientific and medical research is proving that how healthy you are is directly related to how balanced your energy field is.

Bio Electric Field Enhancement is a treatment used to enhance and amplify the body's own ability to heal itself. The BEFE unit produces a "bio charge" compatible with the person stimulating the cell receptors of the body to release toxins and "flush" through the feet, which contain the largest pores. Reported benefits with regular use: pain relief of all forms, allergy relief, blood pressure balance, an increase of energy and vitality, the clearing up of skin conditions, burns healing at an accelerated rate leaving no scarring, and removal of heavy metals and environmental toxins. For more information visit: www.balanceyourstress.com

We bet you can think of dozens of ways to help yourself stay at a positive vibrational frequency. Some very simple suggestions from friends include just walking, gardening, or singing! Lalalalalalala.

Here is a fun exercise in talking to your body! When you're trying to decide whether or not something is right for you, there's an exercise you can do that gives you the right answer every time. It is asking your body. It is really very simple to be in tune with what your body wants for you.

Here's how:

ASK YOUR BODY

Relax, stand straight, legs a bit apart, do not lock your knees, close your eyes and with no expectations, ask your body aloud! "WHICH WAY IS YES?" Pay attention to how your body moves. It may sway forward; it may sway to the right or left. Then ask you body aloud!" WHICH WAY IS NO"? and pay attention to how it moves. Does it sway backward or forward?

Try asking it several times "Which way is yes?" "Which way is no?" until you get consistent movements each time. As a test, you may relax, close your eyes and say, My name is (your name) and ask your body if this is true. See which way it sways. Now put sugar in front of your stomach and ask if the sugar is good for you... now an apple. You can use this method of being in tune with your body whenever you are undecided on a new food or supplement.

Sway muscle-testing http://vst.cape.com/~rch/fox.html on *YouTube*

This is a good place to point out the difference between **IQ** (Intelligence Quotient) and **EQ** (Emotional Quotient). Which one is more important?

Have you ever noticed how some people with high IQs seem to struggle in life, while other happy-go-lucky and not necessarily super-smart people seem to rise to the top? IQ is a number derived from a standardized intelligence test. Some psychologists believe that standard measures of intelligence are too narrow and do not encompass the full range of human intelligence.

EQ, refers to a person's ability to perceive, control, evaluate and express emotions of self and others. Psychologists are suggesting that EQ can play an even more important role in how people fare in life. It is very important to understand that emotional quotient is not the opposite of intelligence quotient; it is not following your heart instead of your head. It is, rather, the beautiful merging of both. People who score high on emotional quotient tests tend to be skilled at interpreting, understanding and acting upon emotions. They are adept at dealing with social or emotional conflicts, expressing their feelings and dealing with emotional situations.

"There is only one corner of the universe you can be certain of improving and that's your own self."
- Aldous Huxley

This is an area where there is always room for improvement. Be self-aware and willing to dig deeper within to learn about yourself. There are several books available on emotional intelligence. One of our favorites is Emotional Intelligence by Daniel Goleman. Another great book, funny and easier to read with a beautiful emphasis on staying connected, is Younger Next Year by Chris Crowley and Henry S. Lodge, M.D.

Steps to integrate into your daily life for Mindfulness

- The moment you wake up, go through a" Gratitude Blast" for 30 seconds naming everything you have to be grateful for. Start with your fingers and toes (if you have them) If not, think of something else.
- Feel the air on your skin – even if you're just walking to the car.
- When you feel upset be aware of where the feeling rests in your body, and keep analyzing the reason for it until you get to a 'core' answer. (I'm afraid, I'm embarrassed, I'm insulted). Realize it's not all that important.
- Know that you are loved. Really.

SELF TEST FOR CHAPTER 6

1. The gastrointestinal tract is sensitive to emotion

a. True

b. False

c. Maybe

2. Vibrational frequency happens

a. On the roller coaster

b. While you're swimming

c. With every thought, word and feeling

3. Your body has a second nervous system that stretches

a. From your hands to your shoulders

b. From your knees to your ankles

c. From your esophagus to your anus

4. Among other benefits, Earthing can normalize cortisol secretion

a. True

b. False

5. Name Five Habits of healthy people

6. Name Three Emotions that cause acidity in the body.

"To hope and dream is not to ignore the practical. It is to dress it in colors and rainbows."

— Anne Wilson Schaef

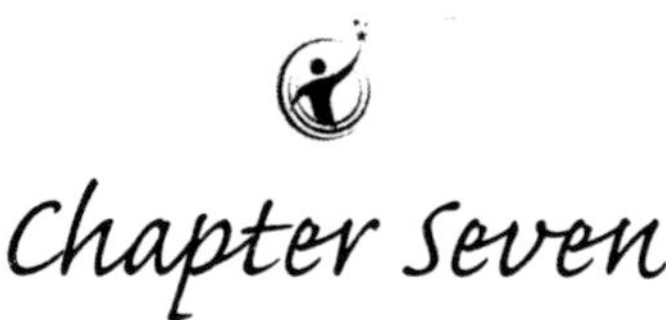

Chapter Seven

THE BEAUTY OF IT ALL

As you may or may not have suspected, a major motivation of both men and women to be healthy is simply this: It Looks Good. Yes, that's right, people who are not feeling well don't really look all that attractive. However, it goes further and lasts longer than just the dark eyes after a night of staying up late and drinking. Chronic inflammation in our body, allergies, fatigue, all make us age faster. Do you seriously want that? Aren't we aging fast enough?

So, because we're so proud of you and the fact that you're going to stay away from foods that make you wrinkle, sag, swell, puff-up, and deteriorate, we're going to give you some great natural food remedies for cosmetic conditions, and some wonderful anti-aging foods to gorge on. Remember, please, to drink 6 – 8 glasses of clean water daily. Vegetable juices and detox teas count towards that daily amount.

You can be Berry Beautiful to a ripe old age by eating your berries! Besides lowering cholesterol, preventing diabetes and cancer and boosting your immunity, they also make your skin glow. Berries are filled with antioxidants, phytochemicals, flavanoids, carotenoids, polyphenols, vitamins and minerals that are all known to benefit the skin. You don't have to know what they are – you just have to eat them. Throw them in your green drink in the morning!

You should know by now that everything we've told you in the previous chapters about drinking water, eating your vegetables, and cleansing will not only keep you healthy – but it will keep you looking great. Your digestion is written all over your face! You know those deep lines some people have running from the sides of their nose to the corner of their lips? The worse your bowel movements are, the deeper those lines are! What about bagginess under the eyes? That's from inflammation in the intestines as well as not having the kidneys nice and flushed. Sagging jowls? That's your stomach crying out for help in digestion. For centuries the Chinese have been able to read the face to treat the body. We can just do it backwards here. Treat the body (kindly) first, and your face will read: Happy... Healthy... Beautiful.

Foods that help us stay young and give us beauty from within all contain high concentrations of the minerals sulfur, silicon, zinc, iron and/or manganese. They all have an alkaline reaction in the body rather than an acidic one (remember we talked about that?) They all have high levels of antioxidants and anti-inflammatory properties.

All fresh, organic, fruits and vegetables are beautifying. However, some especially beautifying foods are:

Aloe Vera	Arugula
Burdock root	Coconuts (& Coconut oil)
Cucumbers	Figs
Hemp Seeds	Macadamia Nuts
Olives (& Olive oil)	Onions
Papaya	Pumpkin Seeds
Radishes	Turmeric
Watercress	Curcumin
Black seeds	Chia & Flax seeds
Sprouts	Sprouted nuts
Fermented foods	

So make sure you're not forgetting these cosmetic collaborators when you prepare your food.

Getting at least 30 minutes a day of sun exposure helps your natural production of Vitamin D which is essential for your bones, muscles and nerves and immune system. You must have your

> **"Cheerfulness and contentment are great beautifiers and are famous preservers of youthful good looks."**
> **- Charles Dickens**

skin exposed to the sun to do this. Getting sun through your office window does not count.

Mindfulness exercises and relaxation techniques are essential for beauty. Have you ever noticed that a truly beautiful person has a relaxed countenance? It doesn't matter how gorgeous your features are if they are all squinted up in a frown. You must be relaxed, calm, serene, mysterious, to look beautiful. This all applies to men as well as women. Your power shines through when you are in a relaxed (ready for anything) state.

Aloe Facial Treatment: For a lovely face lift in 30 minutes, rub aloe gel onto the skin. You will find that the skin seems to be firmer and tighter.

Papaya Facial Treatment: Use a papaya that is almost ripe (about 3/4 ripe). Cut the fruit and rub your face with the fruit. The more unripe the fruit, the stronger the enzymes will be. Make sure the enzymes are not burning around the eyes and lips. Let the fruit soak in for about 5 – 10 minutes. Then wash off thoroughly. This treatment will cleanse and clarify the skin.

Banana Facial Treatment: Mix a half of ripe banana with 1 tsp. of honey and 1 tsp of yogurt. Smear it all over your face and leave it on for 20 minutes before you rinse off with warm water.

For Dry Skin: Massage either olive oil or coconut oil into your skin and allow the oil to soak into the skin for about 20 minutes. Towel off any excess oil.

Ursula's favorite beauty tips:

Coconut Oil Mask: Use equal parts coconut oil and Bob's Red Mill baking soda which is aluminum free. Mix as much as you'll need for a few weeks. The baking soda makes a great natural skin exfoliate because it has a gentle yet course texture. Mix it in a pan and heat it up for 3 – 5 minutes. Put it in a glass container and put it in the freezer for just about 10 minutes so it will bind. Then, use it as a scrub and leave on your face for about 20 minutes. Rinse thoroughly. If you use this mixture each day for 6 days you will be amazed at how miraculously clean and soft your skin is! This mask will help to clear up wrinkles, acne, and brown spots improving the overall appearance of the skin.

Grape Mask: Smash three well-cleansed grapes with a mortar and pestle. (Cleanse them in food grade hydrogen peroxide first). Add 1/2 tablespoon white sugar. Leave on the face and neck for 15 minutes.

Pat's favorite beauty tips: Pat actually worked her way through Acupuncture school as a massage therapist and esthetician. Naturally, she had the latest technology and skin care products at her fingertips. However, it was the natural kitchen-product tips that seemed to nourish both the skin and the soul. Here are some favorite beautifying tricks she shared with her facial clients.

For Brighter Skin: Vitamin C added to the diet is the quickest way to insure a bright complexion. Add a slice of lemon or grapefruit to a jug of water and drink all day! If you want to put your treatment into overdrive, then soak a clean cotton pad with organic orange juice. Wipe it across your face and neck. Then rinse and pat dry. You'll have to do this each day for about a week to see results – but you WILL see results! You just might want to do this each morning or evening before your shower.

For an Instant Face Lift: After you've cleansed your skin, smooth a teaspoon of honey all over your face. After it sets for about a minute, take your fingertips and lightly "drum" them from jaw line to forehead 3 times. Then, let it sit about 10 minutes before rinsing thoroughly with warm water. The honey will act as a drawing agent and pull out skin impurities. It is also a natural moisturizer!

It goes without saying that regular exercise will bring blood and oxygen to your skin which will make you glow! Remember that your tissues heal with a steady supply of blood and oxygen. Now that your blood is going to be filled with a steady supply of nutrients and antioxidants, you will want to make sure it's reaching that pretty face of yours.

To make sure your face is receiving the movement it needs to stay detoxified and vibrant, feel free to take any small amount of oil you have (olive oil, coconut oil, sesame oil) and massage lightly in an upward motion from your neck to your forehead and around your eyes in an inward motion.

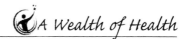

Steps to help integrate into your daily life for Beauty

- Relax
- Use coconut oil in cooking
- Have a small glass of flavored aloe vera each day
- Make yourself a nurturing facial treatment once per week.

Self Test for Chapter Seven

1. Chinese health practitioners can gauge your health by looking at your face.

a. True

b. False

2. Some signs of poor health that we can easily see are

a. Bags or dark circles under the eyes

b. Sagging jowls

c. Deep lines from the nose to the mouth

d. All of the above

5. To help yourself look your best you must

a. Eat fresh organic foods

b. Follow some form of relaxation

c. Make sure you exercise to move your blood & oxygen each day

d.All of the above.

3. Name 5 especially beautifying foods

4. For Dry skin, you can use which of the following

a. Papaya or Banana

b. Honey or Grape

c. Olive Oil or Coconut Oil

"For a long, healthy life, you need
a plan and a purpose.
It could be family, writing a book,
becoming president. Without a purpose,
plan or objective, what do you need?"

— Irving Ladimer, 96

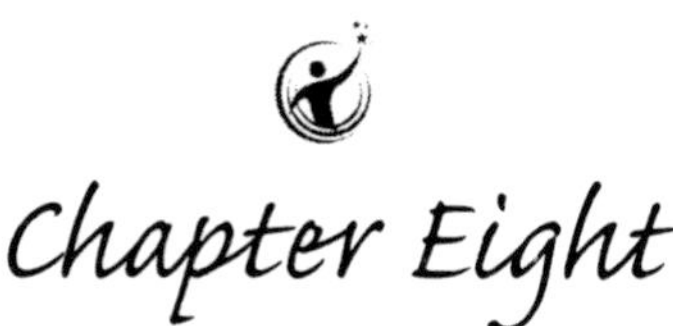

OUR TYPICAL DAYS

We'll start with Pat. She's isn't nearly as self-disciplined as Ursula. It's like comparing... well it's like comparing Italians to Germans. There, I said it. Running a business as a full time health practitioner and having time for her husband keeps Pat pretty busy. She's also Director of the FIOH Naples externship location, and conducts weekend practicals for hypnotherapy students, while continuing her studies in metaphysical sciences and holistic psychology. Add to that the joy of sleepovers from her grandson and frequent flights to see her granddaughter, and you can see that hanging out in the kitchen preparing meals is not always feasible.

Pat prefers to keep her diet simple and fast and clean. Pat's diet is gluten free, GMO free, and for the most part dairy free and soy free. When she has raw foods, she always has some warm tea to help the digestive process. Here she will tell you about her typical day:

I wake up at the same time each morning and have a hot cup of pure water with a wedge of lemon. No more coffee for me. I happily sip on that while I take care of my parrot and check my emails. Weekdays I go for a neighborhood walk. Weekends are usually a bit more intense at the gym. I should probably go to the gym more often, but I'm much more accepting of myself 'as is'. Is there room for improvement? You bet! Am I going to stress about it? No. One day at a time – doing the best I can.

Then I have a small glass of homemade kombucha tea with my probiotic. Thankfully, my husband makes the kombucha tea for me from "starts" that he gets from Ursula! Otherwise, I would be spending a fortune. Before I run out the door for work, I pack my lunch and make myself a juice smoothie in my Nutribullet. I have to admit that my Nutribullet purchase was one of the best decisions I ever made. I haven't juiced this much in 20 years.

I pour this out of the Nutribullet and into my large capped tumbler, stick a straw in, and out the door I go. I sip my green drink slowly on the way to work.

Pat's juice smoothie consists of:

- Raw, organic spinach
- Organic grapes or organic blueberries or organic mangoes
- Chia seeds
- 1 large scoop of Protein powder made from pea protein
- 1 small scoop of L glutamine
- 1 small scoop of diatomaceous earth
- 1 tablespoon liquid gluten free multivitamin
- Pure water to taste

What I bring to work: A small bag of whichever berry or fruit is in season. Grapes, tangerines, blueberries, oranges. I am usually snacking on this about an hour before lunch.

Most days I have at least ½ of a large baked organic sweet potato. I don't need a thing on them... they taste delicious just plain. With my sweet potato, sometimes I have a piece of fish or chicken; sometimes, just greenbeans. (No, I'm not a vegetarian... give me time... I'm getting there).

Sometimes I make myself tuna or chicken salad with vegennaise and have it over a bed of shredded lettuce.

I'm usually not hungry for a snack in the afternoon, but just in case, I keep pistachios and cashews at work (raw and organic). As soon as I get a chance I'm going to get another Nutribullet for the office! I'd love to have an afternoon green drink at work.

I either drink water with lemon or Ginger Ale Kombucha Tea (yum!).

For dinner 3 times a week I have fish or chicken or maybe even a fresh made organic turkey or beef burger along with either salad or green beans or whatever fresh vegetable is in season. (Love my asparagus!) The rest of the time I try to stick to either a brown rice and sautéed vegetable dish, or quinoa and sautéed vegetables. Sometimes, I use gluten-free rice pasta for a comfort food dinner. We grow our own organic kale, bok choy and spinach and I use those greens all the time. An easy, filling meal is to take Trader Joe's gluten free, organic vegetable or chicken stock, add my kale or another green, and heat it up. Great tasting soup.

We are fortunate enough to live within walking distance of both a Whole Foods AND a Trader Joes! My husband and I often walk to Whole Foods and feast off of their salad bar.

Usually I don't have dessert, but if I'm in the mood I have enough choices to keep me happy. Coconut yogurt is delicious, especially on blueberries. Chia seed pudding made with coconut milk is nice (although it requires some forethought and work). Sometimes just nibbling on cocoa nibs does the trick. Mary's Gone Crackers herb crackers with a cup of chamomile tea is a great little "let's stop and smell the roses" break.

Since I've been eating this way I find that I know longer have the cravings I used to have for starches and sweets. I generally kick things up a notch and do my more intense cleanses during 'off season' times from May – October.

And that's it! Life is really simple and easy! Ciao!

Now for Ursula! By nature Ursula is strict and regimented in her diet, but in life she is creative and colorful, thus earning the name *Gypsy* by her peers. Her mother cooked healthy every day with fresh produce from the farmer's market that she shopped for every single day. Ursula's family had fish twice per week, but were mostly vegetarian. Rarely did they have meat in her home because it was so expensive. Today, she still consumes fish, but only once every other week, after reading *Grain Brain* from Dr. Perlmutter as he spoke about the benefits of fish oil. Here we will let Ursula tell you about her typical day:

Now that I am "unofficially retired" my alarm clock is the sunlight. The time varies from day to day and if my body feels tired I lay on my MAS Mat for half an hour for an extra kick of energy. I easily drink 2oz of Liquid Biocell, lemon tea (see recipe on the following page) and a cup of Kombucha. After pouring my tea, I sit on my rocking chair where I meditate for 10 minutes, recite 6 affirmations, and let myself read for a few minutes. I read *St. Theresa's Prayer, The Seven Steps of Effective Prayer*, and a motivational reading called "Don't Quit." I always have some other motivational or spiritual book

Ursula's Lemon Tea Receipe:

One shot glass of herbal tea

One shot glass of freshly juiced lemon

One shot glass of liquid ginger

* Once per week I slice ginger, simmer it for 30 minutes and refrigerate the liquid to use for this receipe

that I am reading and I will indulge in this for about 15 minutes as well. I became committed to my morning routine after being inspired by the book *The Miracle Morning* written by Hal Elrod. This routine gives me both energy and peace for the day ahead. I suggest you find your own morning routine, as it will color your entire day.

All my life it has been a priority to exercise. I am very fortunate to belong to a great fitness center with a variety of classes. My morning continues at the fitness center where I partake in yoga, pilates and power class 3 times per week. I walk the beach for one hour 5 days a week with my friends. After the fitness center I consume an orange, banana and nuts (for protein). For lunch I make a smoothie with kefir, spinach, banana, kale, pineapple, 2 dates, hemp, vegetables (they vary), and a superfood blend (my favorite is *God's Herbs*) or I make a salad. I play golf at least once a week, and tennis three times a week. For snacking during these activities I consume healthy snack bars. My favorite ones include, Oskri's Fig bar and Apricot Almond Bar.

The middle of my day usually consists of research, reading, seminars, webinars or conferences to educate myself even more. I feel the more I learn, the less I know that I know.

If I am home for lunch, I make a juice and/or large salad. If I feel lazy I drink Biotta's Bruess Vegetable Juice and drink it from a wine glass. My salad consists of arugula, mushrooms, kale, beans, tomatoes and other various vegetables for flavor and I add one tablespoon of lemon or lime and *Udo's* oil. At the end of the week I clean out my refrigerator and blend all left over vegetables and salads in a vita mix blender to freeze so that later I can use the content for soup.

For dinner I consume soups or salad with tofu and/or a chipotle vegan burger purchased from Costco (yes, I said it, COSTCO!). I converted recently to a new food religion called pescetarianism which allows me freedom to crave and consume fish. I often meet friends for dinner at my favorite local restaurants, raw vegan cafes, and vegan cafés such as The Loving Hut and the Cider Press Café. I try to buy all organic produce from local farmers markets, health food stores and grocery stores. I do a cell cleanse and liver cleanse once a month. I alkalize my body with the good old-fashioned baking soda remedy every other month (see recipe on the following page); or use the lemon with pineapple drink (see recipe).

The main reason I am so diligent about my research and attend so many seminars is because I am passionate about volunteering to

Baking Soda Alkalizer:

- Use 1 – 2 teaspoons of Bob's Red Mill aluminum free baking soda in water.
- Lemon with pineapple drink: 1 Lemon
- ¼ Pineapple1 cup of coconut water
- Mix all in a blender – It helps to change your pH

help others be and stay healthy. Some would call this life's mission and passion Karma Yoga. Imerman Angels allows me to support other cancer patients that are interested in holistic healing. In Naples, Florida, I meet cancer patients in person to share my story thus giving hope and showing them that there is a future after cancer. Volunteering via phone or in person takes up a good deal of the rest of my day.

I love my life. I am in gratitude every day that I am still here. So, enjoy the moment!

"It is very important to have a widespread curiosity about life."

— Irving Kahn, 106

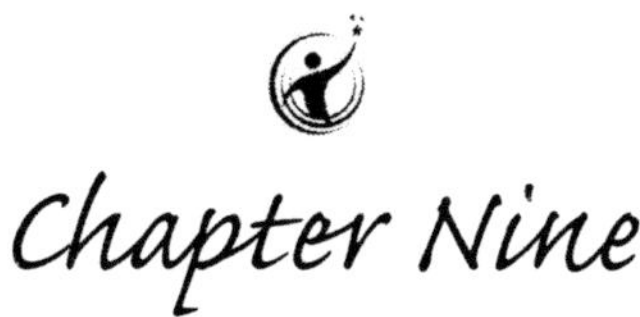

Chapter Nine

SOME ADDITIONAL WISDOM FROM OUR FRIENDS

The articles on the following pages are gifts of knowledge from our esteemed colleagues – for which we are very grateful.

Facts on Fats

by Dee Harris

We have heard for years that fat is bad and increases our risk for heart disease. Also, we have the notion that fat makes us fat. Yes, fat is very concentrated in calories- more than double the calories per gram than carbohydrates or protein. However, that makes them a great source of energy. They also have other important roles in keeping us healthy.

Consider what our body is made of. Our brain is 70 percent fat. Fat also makes up the cell wall of all of our cells so that it protects our precious DNA and energy centers in the cells. Fats moisturize our skin, and are key in regulating the immune system. Fat-soluble vitamins such as vitamin A, E, D and K are critical in body functions and need fat to be absorbed. For example, when you eat a dark green leafy salad, have olive oil in your dressing to help absorb the vitamins. A fat free dressing will sabotage the absorption of key nutrients.

What differentiates good fats versus bad fats is what reduces or drives inflammation. Inflammation is the mother of all disease so; we want to keep our bodies free of inflammation. Omega 3 fatty acids (good fats) such as fish oil and mono-saturated fats such as olive oil help reduce inflammation. Trans fats (bad fats) such as hydrogenated vegetable oils found in many processed foods increases inflammation. Grass fed beef contains Omega 3 fatty acids, so it is less inflammatory than grain fed meats.

There are several categories of fats. Omega 3 and Omega 6 fats are essential because our bodies can't make them, so we need to get them in our diet. Omega 3 fatty acids are found in chia seeds, flax seeds, walnuts, and grass fed meats, and are especially high in fish. Omega 3 fatty acids are anti-inflammatory and need to be in a higher ratio for good health than omega 6 fatty acids. Omega 6 fatty acids include most vegetable oils and grain fed meats. While we need some Omega 6's, our western diet consists of too many Omega 6 and too few Omega 3's.

This imbalance is what causes heart disease and other conditions.

Omega 9 fats are non-essential because our body can make them. They are also called mono-saturated fats. Omega 9s are in olive oil, peanut oil sunflower oil, sunflower, and canola oils, nuts and avocados. Omega 9s do not cause inflammation (unless they are genetically modified or overheated) and can help reduce heart disease risks and other chronic conditions. Omega 9s do not interfere with the Omega 3 to 6 ratio and, if used instead of omega 6, can actually help improve the Omega 3 ratio.

As mentioned, hydrogenating the vegetable oils to trans fats is a contributor to poor health. Mostly found in processed foods and fast foods, it is well documented that trans fats (oil turned into a stable hard fat), clogs the arteries. This is far worse than saturated fat found in meats. In 2006, the FDA mandated manufacturers to list trans fats on the nutritional facts label. However, it isn't enough because it still allowed for less than ½ gram of trans fats to be in the product and be labeled "No Trans-Fats". So you could still be getting trans fats without even knowing it. It's all in the fine print now. Beware of ingredients saying partially hydrogenated oil.

We can actually create unhealthy oils in our own kitchen. By heating oil to a high "smoke point", we can degrade a healthy oil and cause oxidation and toxic fumes. Beware of smoking oils and don't cook oils to a high temperature. Certain oils lend themselves to cooking at higher temperatures. Here is a link to an easy chart for smoke points: http://bit.ly/1obKzNI

When purchasing oils, make sure they are not from a genetically modified source. For example, corn and soy are the most genetically modified foods. Canola oil is also genetically modified and highly processed and should be avoided.

Coconut oil, although a plant saturated fat, is a very healthy fat and does not contribute to heart disease. It is a medium chain triglyceride oil. It is easily digested and a powerful fuel for the brain. In fact, it is used as a therapeutic treatment in brain disorders such as Alzheimer's. It is also an antimicrobial so it helps our immune system rid us of pathogenic agents.

So how can you get the right balance of healthy fats into your daily life? Avoid processed and fast food. Start out with buying only organic oils. Eat wild fish at least three times per week. Eat organic nuts and seeds daily. If you eat red meat, eat grass fed beef only (not grain fed). Use extra virgin olive oil. Use coconut oil in cooking daily or use MCT oil and mix it with your extra virgin olive oil. Follow the smoke point guide and don't overheat your oils. Consider taking a high quality omega 3 supplement.

Because fats are concentrated in calories, be aware of portion sizes. The average size of a nut serving is 1/8th of a cup and 1-2 teaspoons of seeds. 1 teaspoon of butter and oil is a serving. ½ of an avocado is a serving. Aim for 8 teaspoons of oil or butter and 4 servings of nuts and seeds per day. When we supersize our fat portions, even if it is a healthy fat, we may start to store more fats. This is especially true if you are also eating a diet high in carbohydrates.

Therefore, the key is a low carbohydrate, higher healthy fat diet.

Dee Harris, *RD, LDN, CDE*
D-Signed Nutrition, LLC
27499 Riverview Center Blvd., Suite 214
Bonita Springs, FL 34134
Mobile: 239-404-0879
Office: 239-444-4204 ext. 111
www.D-SignedNutrition.com
info@d-signednutrition.com

Challenges & Opportunities

by Dr. Nancy Vance

"The greatest mistake in the treatment of diseases is that there are physicians for the body and physicians for the soul, although the two cannot be separated." — Plato

Body, mind and soul - a simple phrase that has endless implications. Great teachers throughout our history have encouraged us to turn inward and attend to the mind, the body and the spirit. Yet, most of us remain engaged in an outer world filled with personal, financial, business, political and even world stress. We are in a constant state of 'out of time, out of money and out of touch.' Too often we will find that the answer culminates with words on a prescription pad. We have forgotten the answer that lies within. Prescriptions come with a high cost and I am not referring to insurance you buy or amount of cash you hand across the counter. I am referring to a much higher cost. In our rush to relieve our suffering, we inadvertently but frequently abandon the concept of cure. We are comfortable with "management" of disease accepting the inevitable dependence on an increasing number of prescription medications. Our minds never wonder back to the cause of our affliction. We experience only acceptance and perhaps gratitude that suffering is relieved while we return to our outer world. Ah, but it is the relief of that suffering that allows disease to progress...

The body, the mind and the spirit are intricately connected and disruption in the balance (homeostasis) of one will certainly be reflected in the other. Have you used or heard the phrase, "It is hurtful to the soul"? An experience that is "hurtful to the soul" has obvious implications to the mind but consider the effects on the body as well. Stress hormones are elevated, while repair hormones are depressed. Indeed, a cascade of events is unleashed upon the body. Blood is shunted away from the gut where greater than 70% of our immune system resides. Of course, absorption of nutrients is then impaired and we are unable to absorb the nutrients necessary to create adequate serotonin and neurotransmitter balance critical for a healthy mood (mind). But remember, we also need those nutrients for vital processes such as DNA repair, detoxification, cellular function and new cell production. That blood that is shunted away from the gut is driven to the heart, lungs and extremities in the "flight or fight" response that once served us well in times of danger. Now, in our world of constant stress, it results in elevated blood pressure, heart disease, chronic gastrointestinal distress – ultimately leading to all forms of chronic disease.

Of grave concern is the prevalence of chronic disease as it now accounts for 7-in-10 deaths in the United States. While nearly half of all adults live with more than one chronic disease, the percentage of children with chronic disease is escalating. Of course, in our current medical model we are quick to respond. A pill for your blood pressure, a proton pump inhibitor for your stomach, antibiotics for infection the immune system failed to prevent, an anxiety pill and an antidepressant for the imbalance in your neurotransmitters, a pill to help you sleep as melatonin is not being created, and on I can go... We do have a pill for every ill. But did we fix or even identify the cause? Symptoms are the body's warning system. Did we heed the warning or did we quiet it? An honest look at our medical model shows great advances in quantity of life but frequently it fails to offer quality of life. We have moved to a strict system model where we care for the cancer in Room 2, the hypertension in Room 1, and the joint pain in Room 3. We no longer look at the patient as a whole but as a laundry list of complaints. This is a medical model where time is priority and it is measured by the physician, the patient, and the insurance company as well as the government. It is a model of ever increasing protocols designed to take the physician and the patient out of the equation. Lost is the concept of cause. Without identification of the cause, however, we can never expect a cure.

To achieve good health we must return to the balance that the body, mind and spirit require.

We face many obstacles. We must first address the stress that is placed upon us and we place upon ourselves. Stress management must be a priority as stress is associated with every chronic disease. It can and should be measured though it is not commonly done in traditional medicine. We may even predict survival in cancer and disease progression based upon the stress hormone cortisol. We have many tools that include nutrition, herbs, exercise, laughter, music, and meditation. We must provide our bodies with minerals, nutrients, proteins that are required to detoxify, repair and rebuild. With 25 million new cells produced each second, we have a high demand for those nutrients. Yet, the average person is, in fact, over fed and undernourished with close to 500 calories per day coming from sugar or high fructose corn syrup (HFCS). This is a condition that, in reality, further depletes the body of nutrients as vitamins and minerals must be stolen from other bodily functions to process this elevated load in sugar. Our reliance on processed foods further leaves us depleted of the vital nutrients resulting in poor repair mechanisms and an inability to respond to the stresses of our environment – a recipe for disease. Even the medications we so cherish for relief of our symptoms result in further depletions of nutrients. Of course, an even greater threat to our limited resources is the multitude of toxins that we are exposed to on a daily basis. These toxins found in our air, in our home, and on our food are an often unacknowledged component of our environment that have a large role in the development and progression of disease.

This toxic burden further increases our need for nutrients and antioxidants to combat the ongoing damage that we incur.

All is not lost. Our challenges appear overwhelming but so are our opportunities. We can measure those very nutrients that our body requires and we can replace them. We can measure and repair the damage that stress wreaks upon our body. Most fascinating, we now live in an age where we have sequenced the entire genome. Knowledge of our own specific DNA allows us to assess our relative risk for certain diseases and modify our environment accordingly. Perhaps even greater importance lies in the research on the cellular process of methylation as it has such wide reaching implications and offers greater insight into our internal environment. For those with open eyes, before us lie many opportunities to strengthen our mind and our spirit as well as our body.

Ultimately, we clearly have the right, the responsibility, and the means to control our environment and our health. Knowledge is, indeed, not only powerful but essential. We must maintain an awareness of our internal and external environment. We must nourish our souls as well as our bodies. We must have gratitude for the opportunities we have to guide our health and our future. We live in an information age that allows us freedom to explore our own healthy paths. While traditional medicine is imperfect, it has given us an expectation of a longer life and there will likely come a time when we are grateful for the comfort and care it offers. Yet, our own goal should remain to delay our entry into that system by maintaining our own health in the manner in which it evolved to thrive. It is through this balance in all forms with attention to the spirit as well as the body that true health resides.

Nancy Vance, *MD, FAARFM*
Insight to Health & Wellness, Inc.
www.Insight2HW.com

Energy Medicine... the Future

by Richard Campagnalia

On September 30th, 2007, I had a terrible auto accident where I almost lost my right foot. As a result of that injury my life has changed and so have my view points on energy.After two surgeries and chronic pain I started my research on ways to alleviate pain. Two things I came up with were laser therapy and pulsed electromagnetic frequencies (PEMF). At that point I purchased my first laser and my first PEMF device, which within a two month period relieved my pain and got me walking normally again. My experience with these devices prompted me to open up my clinic Holistic Solutions where we use energy technologies to help heal the body of different traumas.

Pulsed Electro-magnetic Field (PEMF) activates electrically charged particles in ways that stimulate healing in the body. When Dr. Oz saw this technology he exclaimed, "Today we are changing the practice of medicine." Physicians have long known that "the body electric" is for real. Tiny electric currents and magnetic fields are constantly firing off inside you. Pulsating electromagnets produce invisible energy waves that increase blood flow and normalize some electrical impulses to, and in, nerves. Your nerves, cartilage, muscles and blood all rely on a symphony of dancing ions.

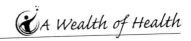

ENERGY

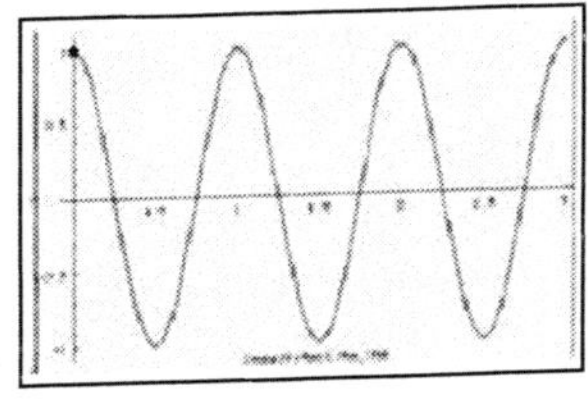

All life is energy. Every nerve impulse in your body is an electric current. Every cell in your body is a mini-battery pumping out 70-90 millivolts - when healthy. Our muscles are powered by chemical energy. The food that you eat is really just fuel for the fire. Eating is like throwing coal in a furnace. Digestion is nothing more than a slow form of burning that produces energy for your body to live on. In fact, death itself is defined as the absence of electrical activity in the brain. In the end, all life is Energy. If you optimize that energy, you optimize your health. If you charge your body with the right frequencies, you prevent disease. The proper use of energy in the healing arts has a long and significant history: from the TENS machines and laser surgery to the use of sound waves to break up kidney stones, or X-rays and magnetic fields to see into the body to the use of light to clean the blood. Some forms of energy are more effective than others.

The Nature of Energy

All of the energy that we normally think of is characterized by both particle and wavelike properties. The waveform of all these energies can be graphed as a hertzian wave (either in the form of a sine wave or a step wave).

We're talking about everything from electricity to magnetism, from light to sound. The only difference between all of these forms of energy is how fast the waves rise and fall (the frequency) and how intense those rises and falls are (their amplitude).

SCALAR ENERGY

Scalar energy, however, is a different animal. Understand, scalar energy has always existed - since the beginning of time - however, it's only recently that scientists have discovered and begun to make use of it. It was actually back in the mid 1800's that the existence of scalar energy was first proposed in a series of 4 groundbreaking equations by the Scottish mathematician, James Clerk Maxwell.

$$\nabla \times H = \varepsilon_0 \, \delta E/\delta t + J$$
$$\nabla \times E = -\mu_0 \, \delta H/\delta t$$
$$\nabla \; H = 0$$
$$\nabla \; E = \rho/\varepsilon_0$$

Don't even think about trying to understand these equations.

- Just as a minor reference, H refers to the magnetic field. E refers to the energy field. Most of the other symbols are Greek letters such as epsilon and delta. The upside down triangle represents the Vector Differential.

But forget all of that. The key to these equations - what makes them remarkable history is the use of the ρ symbol, which stands for Scalar Charge Density - thus representing the first time that the existence of scalar energy was theoretically proposed.

It was almost a half-century later before Nicola Tesla actually was able to demonstrate the existence of scalar energy. When Tesla died, he took the secret of scalar generation with him, and it took almost another full century before science was once again able to positively demonstrate the existence of scalar energy and turn to an exploration of its potential.

What are Scalar Waves? The standard definition of scalar waves is that they are created by a pair of identical (or replicant) waves (usually called the wave and its antiwave) that are in phase spatially, but out of phase temporally. That is to say, the two waves are physically identical, but 180° out of phase in terms of time. The net result is that scalar waves are a whole different animal from normal hertzian waves. They even look different - like an infinitely projected mobius pattern on axis.

Different – How?

Scalar energy is different from standard hertzian electromagnetic fields in a number of important ways.

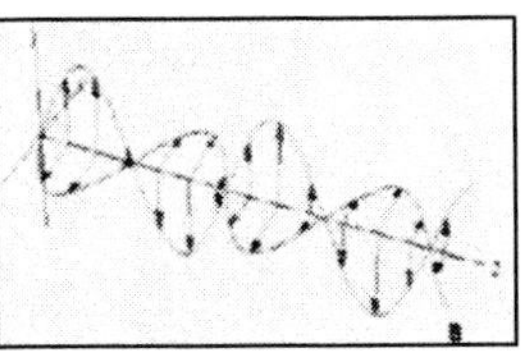

- First, it's more field like than wavelike. Instead of running along wires or shooting out in beams, it tends to "fill" its environment. This becomes very important in terms of developing the technology for embedding products with scalar energy.

- For many of the same reasons, it is capable of passing through solid objects with no loss of intensity. In fact, that is exactly what Tesla demonstrated over 100 years ago when he projected a scalar wave through the earth with no loss of field strength. Again, this is vital in the development of technology capable of embedding scalar energy in products.

- It implants its signature on solid objects. This is actually the heart of the issue. All electric fields can implant their signature on objects, but not to the degree that scalar energy can. This becomes extremely important when we actually talk about the mechanics of embedding the energy field in products, and then transferring that charge from the products into every cell of your body.

- Scalar energy can regenerate and repair itself indefinitely. This also has important implications for the body. In other words, once the charge is implanted, you can keep it there with the regular ingestion of charged products.

- In fact, the right scalar frequencies have a whole range of profound beneficial effects on the human body.

- In the New Age community there has been much talk of the benefit of things like Tachyons, Radionics, and Pyramids, etc. Analysis shows that these are all, at heart, scalar generating devices - but cannot come close to the effectiveness of ingesting scalar enhanced products.

For more information on products with scalar energy visit:
www.holistic-healthsolutions.com

Healthy Eating

by Tania Melkonian

The decision to live consciously and healthfully - including the pursuit of eating well - seems to come with the burden of due diligence. How do we eat healthy? One source says X food is great for our hearts. Another says it is terrible for our blood sugar and that it is better to eat Y. The whole process becomes confusing not to mention full of displeasure. We even use language like 'I was good all week but on Saturday, I cheated and had a slice of pizza/wine/ice cream/ chocolate/popcorn.' There is guilt and stigma attached to one's food choices that accompany the onslaught of contradictory information. It is no wonder then, that after a brief investigation of how to eat healthy, we throw up our hands and give up entirely or surrender to fads and modes of eating. We say to ourselves 'If I just become a vegan/Paleo devotee/ macro-biotic eater/raw food-ist, I will definitely be eating healthy'. Entry into these dietary clubs comes at a price. We box ourselves in so tightly to conform to these labels and we ignore the healthy effect on our souls of enjoying our experience of eating.

Additionally, if our ethnic lineage features a certain food or food group which our new club does not (a South or South-East Asian person becoming a Paleo devotee and relinquishing rice, to offer a caricature example); we ignore the contribution that tradition and culture make to our emotional health as well as the anthropological significance of food. If we do make decisions based on what we read or hear, they are not organic. We approach the question so intellectually, rather than viscerally, that we tend to adopt a 'more is better' attitude. Then, we hear people talking about eating 'just a giant salad' for lunch. None of us should be eating 'giant' anything. We restrict and limit ourselves so stridently that we lose our sense of what we really need. Instead of eating clean - real food that includes lots of plants - and allowing our palates and stomachs to recalibrate, we fill every little available space with what we have read is healthy until we cannot feel the difference between satiety and being stuffed.

We can distill a few basic, un-confusing truths from the mash of noise that comes at us!

Vegetables are good for everyone. Processed foods are bad for everyone. Beyond that, it is hard to say what is good or bad for each individual. Let us be guided by the more nuanced areas of the issue. Let us be guided by our tastes, our personal, physiological and ethnic constitutions and by our social circumstances. And let us not stuff ourselves (even if it is at an all-you-can-eat salad bar) because more is NOT better!

Why is processed food bad? The most resounding answer is in the liver. The liver is like the attic of the body storing anything that is not of immediate use or whose use it does not recognize. So, anything synthetic, denatured or processed is not recognizable to the body and gets stored in the liver. Just as the stuff we store in our attics becomes clutter, so too does the unrecognizable matter in the liver. In fact, that clutter eventually takes the easily storable form of fat. A fatty congested liver has a domino effect on all the systems of the body making even the useable nutrients that we take in, difficult or even impossible to access for healing and growth. Extend this principle of liver storage logically and it means that even real unprocessed foods that have preservatives and other additives is going to end up stored indefinitely in the liver.

Why are vegetables good for everyone? If inflammation is the enemy of the body then discouraging or undoing that inflammation is the most healing and/or preventative action we can take. The phytonutrients contained in vegetables will help us with those processes. More importantly, every single culture has included vegetables, raw (later cooked) and wild (later cultivated) in its cuisine. It is the living part of a plate. Vegetables lend the brightness to food in taste, color and story!

Why should we always be a little bit hungry? Moving through functional life in an agitated, hurried way, we miss moments. The opposite of this energy is meditation. In meditation, we stop to simply be instead of do. There is plenty of science behind the assertions that meditation initiates a relaxation response in the body that turns on healing and restoration and takes us out of that survival reflex. Eating until satisfied - but not full - is the eating equivalent of meditation. Eating slowly and just until satiety but with a little room allows for the same exploration for the needs of the physical body that breathing slowly and meditating provides for the subtle bodies (mind and spirit). When we eat to fullness, we behave desperately as if the continued existence of our bodily tissues require an immediate and excessive stream of nutrients. Leaving a little room gives our digestive system a buffer as well as our appetites a chance to be curious!

So we should ALL eat real, unprocessed food that includes vegetables... and not too much of it. Beyond that, it is true that some of us should have only plants. Some people have difficulty digesting grains, are allergic to nuts, experience spikes in blood sugar with too much fruit, find the texture of beans unappetizing, feel that eating animal flesh is unethical, or simply don't like brussell sprouts!! The way we come to know where we are on the very long spectrum that lies in between vegetables on one end and processed food on the other is by **eating clean**. That includes - but is not limited to - eating hormone-free, organic non-genetically modified food. It also means accepting, graciously, food that has been prepared with love, even if it features foods that might not be part of your regular 'diet'. Unless you are physically sensitive or allergic a little grain or dairy or caffeine or even sugar offered say, at a celebration or in community, will not undo any other well-intentioned behavior. In fact, accepting the generosity with an equally generous spirit will flood the body with endorphins that cultivate a healing response rather than a stressful one. It means eating without guilt and shame to pollute the experience. We don't 'deserve' a cookie because we had our daily wheatgrass shot. We deserve to experience fully, everything we do with mindfulness. It includes a respect for our ancestral predecessors who helped us to understand what it meant to be human one or two or more generations ago. They gave us perspective on how cultural cuisines evolved as extensions of peoples' relationships with earth's bounty. Quieting all the noise and really listening for all these cues makes the journey to eating healthy. Eat real food that includes lot of vegetables. Then eat clean. And listen!

Tania Melkonian
Co-founder EATomology!
www.EATomology.com.

Creating Permanent Change – Sustainable Solutions – Balance!

by Jamie L. Kliewe

Weight Loss • Disease Prevention • Anti-Aging
Organic • GMO's • Pharmaceuticals • Diabetes
Pre-Diabetes • Heart Disease • Cancer!
Vegan • Paleo • Mediteranian • Aryuvedic
South Beach • Atkins • Grain / No Grain
Gluten • Sugar • Diet • Health!

AAAHHHH! What does all this mean to me?

We have been inundated with lots of great information about how to live a healthy and disease-free life.

We have all received good advice throughout our lives that had great potential to really make an impact on our health and vitality. We have good intentions about making changes that last. We've read about the latest diet craze and thought "Yea, I'm going to do it this time". We all have day dreams of the perfect body, the perfect eating habits, the perfect energy level to go out and conquer the world. We've made a pact with ourselves over and over again that this time it will be different. However, we often find ourselves frustrated and feeling defeated because with the best of intentions we still come up short.

We look at all the information available about health and disease prevention and most of it is confusing and contradictory at best. Will a pill actually cause us to lose 30lbs in a week without changing out lifestyle? Should I eat meat? Not eat meat? Grains or no Grains? But I don't like Kale – at all. Is sugar really all that bad? Does diet soda count as water? Is McDonalds really that unhealthy? I can't afford to eat Organic. I have no time to cook healthy. Ok, I can do this. It's been a week and I don't see any results. You know what, screw it. I can't do this. I feel lousy. There has to be a better way. Maybe I'll try this new diet, looks like it might be easier. Not again. I've been at this for two weeks and still nothing. Actually I feel worse. Maybe it's just hopeless.

If you have ever found yourself having this dialog you are not alone. The world of healthy eating has gotten very confusing for most of us. We are being overpowered with the latest diet regimes and the newest pills that claim to solve our issues with weight, energy, disease, and many other issues that we face. So, how exactly do we get on with the task of eating and living healthy? What is healthy anyway?

Let's discuss some ways to create long lasting and sustainable changes in our lives that will have a powerful impact on us and our families. First off, we need to realize that it took us a long while to get here. In other words, whatever our situation is with our health, this did not happen overnight. It has been years of habitual behavior that has been become ingrained in our lives and most of us work on auto pilot.

We have been taught certain eating habits and lifestyle regimes based on inaccurate, politically and money driven information. We've listened to commercials, read the claims on packaging and been taught the USDA guidelines about diet and took it all as the definitive and accurate source on how to live a health and disease free life. So all these years later many are realizing that most of it has not been accurate at all. So where do we go from here? We need to retrain ourselves and our society based on the facts. How do we do that? Let's go over some tips.

Tip 1) Be patient – this is going to be a process of learning a new way of life. We must gradually retrain ourselves about what is healthy. This will not be an overnight affair.

Tip 2) Allow for setbacks – As with any new adventure there is a learning curve. We are not going to ever be perfect. In the beginning there may be some frustrating moments, but that's ok. Know that. Expect that. Keep going.

Tip 3) Don't try to build Rome in a day – Pick one or two things you are going to make a commitment to change. Do those things consistently for at least two to three weeks until it becomes part of your daily routine without much thought. Then once you have that down pick a few more things and do the same.

Tip 4) If it's not working change it – we are all different and we can't expect that what works for one person is going to be a great fit for someone else. It's ok to try something new.

Tip 5) Give yourself permission to go bad – Yes, I said it. We are never going to be perfect so we might as well put away the sledge hammer and go easy on ourselves. Using the 80/20 or I like the 90/10 rule which is 10 or 20 percent of the time you get to indulge in something bad. If we give ourselves permission instead of beating ourselves up over it, most of the time the need to go "bad" turns into a small treat instead of night of binge eating.

Tip 6) Meditate on what it is you really desire in terms of your health. Maybe write it down in a journal. Often times we think of vague images or unrealistic pictures of what we really want as far as our health is concerned. Are you more concerned with looks, feeling well, disease prevention? What does that look like for you? Everyone is different and to get this down on paper may be a great way to get this image clear. We may have some short term desires and long term desires. Let's get it in focus!

Tip 7) Get Help – there is so much information available to us and it can be so darn confusing as to what we should be doing. Keep it simple. If you don't know ask. Join a group if you can or get with a Health Coach to educate you. Find like minded people to communicate with. Doing this alone will only isolate you and cause you to get frustrated and most likely will result in throwing in the towel. Find people through network groups, community groups or start your own group to help build a support team. We don't have to do this alone.

Tip 8) Take small Steps forward – The key here is to not put ourselves in a state of overwhelm to which we say, just screw it. I can't do this. Learn one new thing a week about healthy living. Pick one topic and look into it and see if you can implement it into your life.

Tip 9) Get Back on the Horse – If you fall – Get Back Up! When learning to walk (though we may not remember this activity) it was a series of getting up and falling down. This is the same process when learning something new. It's okay to fall down, but we must get back up!

Tip 10) Have Fun! – We have to make this enjoyable. Treat yourself kindly! Be your own best friend. If you were giving advice to your best friend what would it be? Take that advice. Often times we know what we would say to someone else that would be kind and supportive but with ourselves we do a bit of slicing and dicing. Pick some fun activities that you enjoy and work them into your schedule. You deserve it!

I wish you all the best. Never give up on yourself!

Jamie L. Kliewe, *LMT, NCTMB, CMLDT, COE*
Certified Holistic Health Coach
Mind Body and Soul Holistic Wellness Center
Central Ave #305
Naples FL 34102
239-234-1608850
www.MBSHWC.com

Your Diet and Your Immune System

by Katherine Ortiz PA-C, MMS, AHAAHP

Many people have sensitivities to many different foods but do not even realize it. They may think they are just tired for no reason or they have difficulty losing weight. Food sensitivities are quite different from true food allergies. In traditional food allergies you get the classic symptoms of hives, rash, difficulty breathing, tongue swelling etc. These are usually immediate reactions and can be life threatening. Food sensitivities are mediated by the immune system just as in food allergies but are mediated by a different immunoglobin called IgG- which is delayed hypersensitivity. If someone ingests a food such as gluten, and they are sensitive to it, the reaction can sometimes be up to 12 hrs. later.

Most sensitivities produce symptoms of fatigue, bloating, gas, acid reflux, chronic migraines, constipation, and inability to lose weight. Other diseases prompted by food sensitivities are autoimmune diseases such as rheumatoid arthritis. The reason behind all this is because food sensitivities create an inflammatory reaction within the body and release toxic cytokine (inflammatory reactants). Also in the small intestine, the foods interact with the lumen (the inner lining of the intestine) and cause an antigen-antibody complex and irritate the lining and this can lead to leaky gut syndrome. Leaky gut syndrome is when the cells in the stomach (enterocytes) create gap junctions, and actual food particles leak out through this barrier when they are not supposed to. This throws the body into an autoimmune reactive state. These antigen-antibody complexes reacted with the body's immune system and create chronic inflammation and stress in the body.

The bacterial toxins in the gut attach to the immune system and produce inflammatory substances such as IL-6, and TNF alpha which also hinder metabolism and create insulin resistance, and therefore cause weight gain. Some people with leaky gut syndrome caused by food sensitivities have chronic weight gain despite healthy eating and exercise. These are the people that truly say they eat healthy and exercise and get no results. There was a study published in 2007 in the journal *Diabetes* in which they performed a complex study on how leaky gut begins, how food sensitivities can lead to chronic inflammation and inflammatory cytokines and prevent fat burning. It was shown that with processed foods, foods high in sugar, and trans fats created an imbalance of good and bad bacteria in the gut which is called dysbiosis. When the lining of the gut is inflamed, junctions open between the tight cells making up the gut walls this is called leaky gut syndrome, these semi-permeable holes in the gut's lining allow bacteria and partially-digested food molecules to slip out into the bloodstream, where they are considered foreign invaders. The immune system attacks full force and white blood cells rush to surround the offending particle and systemic inflammation begins.

I'm not talking about a sore throat or cough. I'm talking about a hidden, smoldering fire created by the immune system as it tries to fight off a daily entourage of food allergies. This kills the good bacteria, the less of the good bacteria leads to overgrowth of the bad intestinal bacteria which promotes weight gain and inflammation. The outward symptoms are bloating, gas, acne, fatigue, sometimes body rashes.

It is important to maintain healthy gut flora with high quality probiotics and whole foods. Also fermented foods such as kefir and sauerkraut have good bacteria to replenish the gastrointestinal tract. It is important to pay attention to your body and what it is doing. If you are having issues with skin rashes, weight gain, bloating, fatigue, or chronic migraines it is important to consider food sensitivities as the root cause of these symptoms. Even if you are eating healthy the foods that are the best for us (we think) could be causing a chronic inflammatory reaction within our gut causing your body to react. The testing is relatively easy and consists of blood work.

Katherine Ortiz *PA-C, M.M.S, AHAAHP*
Fellowship trained in Anti-Aging and Functional Medicine (A4M)
www.Naplesdnawellness.com

Chapter Ten

STOCKING UP FOR SIMPLE RECIPES

We have picked out some of the easiest and most cost effective recipes and ideas in our basket of goodies to share with you. There are PLENTY of great recipes on the internet. Just start googling inexpensive health food recipes and you will find a wide array of information. You know enough now to stay away from the unhealthy ingredients. If you don't have the internet, then we bet you could find a recipe book that is perfect for you at your library or bookstore. Check out the resource section (next chapter) and thumb through a few of our favorite books.

SHOPPING

You would be amazed at what you can find in major grocery chains and mega shopping warehouses. Food items that are organic and also gluten-free are there if you take the time to look. Of course, you'll still have to be sure you're not buying something that is loaded with hydrogenated vegetable oil or corn syrup, but remember this is a learning process. The first time you go to shop with your new standards just give yourself some extra time to read the labels. If you find when you get home that you've bought something - well – poison – just chalk it down to a lesson learned and don't buy it again. If you have the time and energy, most places will let you return those items.

Storage: Pat's husband made her some open shelves above the kitchen sink that are now filled with glass jars for all of her nuts and seeds and fresh spices. She got all the matching glass jars by saving the ones that her Ghee came in when she gave up butter. Make it easy on yourself! All of the milks used (Flaxseed, coconut, hemp) can stay in the cabinets until they are opened because they come in cardboard containers.

In order to keep your momentum going, you'll want your pantry to contain the following staples. Not all at once, of course... but over time, stock up. If you have all these on hand, you'll be whipping up incredibly delicious healthy meals in no time.

Miscellaneous: Baking supplies, condiments

- Vegennaise
- Organic ketchup
- Organic mustard
- Sesame oil
- Extra virgin olive oil
- Coconut Milk, Almond Milk or Rice Milk (refrigerate after opening)
- Vinegar
- Turbniado sugar from natural cane
- Organic pure maple syrup
- Agave nectar
- Organic vegetable broth
- Organic beef broth
- Organic chicken broth
- Dried shredded coconut
- Raw organic honey

Canned Goods

- Wild Planet Wild Sardines in extra virgin olive oil
- Wild Planet Wild Albacore Tuna
- Pineapple chunks in their own juice (not syrup)
- Artichoke Hearts
- Hearts of Palm
- Sundried tomatoes
- Tomato sauce
- Diced tomatoes
- Stewed tomatoes
- Tomato Paste
- Black Olives
- Black Beans
- Red Beans
- Vita Coco pure coconut water

Grains, Pastas, Cereals

- Organic brown rice pasta
- Organic Muesli
- Basmati brown rice
- Earthy Choice 100% Whole Grain Quinoa
- Triple Nut Cereal
- Toasted Oatmeal flakes
- Hemp Plus Granola

Snacks, Nuts, Dried Fruits

- Snacks, Nuts, Dried Fruits
- Sliced almonds
- Cashews
- Pistachios
- Pecans
- Raisins
- Dried fruit like plums or prunes
- Mary's Gone Crackers herb crackers
- Nut Thins
- Terra Chips
- Crunchmaster Multigrain Crackers –oven baked, gluten free
- Coastal Berry Blend: cashews, almonds, cranberries, yogurt chips and wild blueberries (for breakfast on the go)
- Wild Garden Hummus Dip (24 single serving packs – easy to take along)

Seeds

- Chia seeds
- Sunflower seeds
- Pumpkin seeds
- Flax seed

Refrigerator

- Acai superfood juice
- POM Pomegrante juice
- Aloe Vera Juice
- Organic carrot juice (bottled)

* Make sure that there are no sugar or sugar substitutes added

- Kombucha tea
- Organic Greek yogurt
- Made in Nature Dried and unsweetened Figs
- Golden-pitted dates
- Mandarin organs
- Apples
- Pears
- Lemons
- Ginger
- Avocados
- Real Lemon squeezed lemon juices
- Any fresh fruit in season
- Raw cacao nibs
- Ghee (instead of butter)
- Butter (only organic)
- Organic, free range eggs (omega 3)
- Garlic bulbs
- Sweet potatoes

Freezer

- Frozen Fruit such as cherries, blueberries, raspberries, strawberries
- Frozen organic and/ or gluten free waffles
- Frozen organic vegetables such as green beans, broccoli, spinach, peas
- Frozen organic and/ or gluten free burger buns
- Frozen Vegetable burgers

Fish: Make sure it is wild caught, not farmed.

- Wild caught Sockeye Salmon
- Flounder
- Mahi Mahi
- Snapper, Grouper
- Morningstar veggie sausage patties
- Trident Wild Pacific Salmon Burgers
- Cox's East Coast Wild Shrimp
- Bayside Bistro flounder Fillets (wild caught, all natural, breaded)
- Free-range organic chicken
- Grass fed organic beef
- Organic ground turkey

With the these listed ingredients, you can easily make yourself breakfast, lunch or dinner on the fly.

For breakfast, you'll want a little protein, whether it is in the form of animal protein (*i.e.* an egg) or strictly vegetable protein (smoothie). Either one will keep you full until lunchtime. If having eggs, we recommend having them with some sautéed spinach or kale.

BREAKFAST

Easy: A green drink Just blend your spinach, kale or other green with some seeds and fruit and maybe some protein powder. Done.

A little harder: Blend the following for a smoothie:

- Kiefer/yogurt
- One banana
- _ pineapple sliced
- Turmeric Powder
- Spinach and/or kale
    - For protein, add Brazil nuts and/or dates
- Chia seeds
- 3 tablespoons hemp hearts
- Coconut water for the base.

Moderate: Raw spinach or kale with an egg An extremely easy recipe is to place your raw kale or spinach in a frying pan with just a touch of olive oil, butter or ghee. Wait just a few minutes for it to sauté, and then crack an egg over it. Delicious. If you want, serve on some gluten free bread.

Weekend impress company or family recipe: Vegan Pumpkin Coconut Pancakes. In the blender combine:

- 1 cup almond milk or coconut milk
- _ cup pumpkin puree
- _ cut steel cut rolled oats
- _ cut unsweetened shredded coconut
- 3 tablespoons ground flaxseed
- 1 teaspoon ground cinnamon
- Pinch of salt

Puree ingredients in the blender. Cook on a medium-high griddle. They take a little longer than traditional pancakes to be done, so after you flip, turn heat to medium to avoid burning. Serve with a drizzle of maple syrup (the pancakes are unsweetened, but a little maple syrup makes it taste just right).

LUNCH

Easy: Veggie smoothie with kale, carrots, apple, chia seeds, protein powder.

Have sardines on gluten nut thin crackers for a side dish

Moderate: Tuna or Salmon Salad on spinach with black olives, seeds and/or nuts and a baked sweet potato on the side.

Weekend Impress Company or family recipe: Homemade veggie burger. Combine...

- _ chopped onions
- 1 cup adzuki beans
- One cup brown rice cooked
- _ cup garbanzo flour
- Salt, parsley, sage, rosemary, thyme

Mix all ingredients together; add a little water to form burger

Have pan on middle-high heat

Use organic olive oil if necessary

DINNER

Easy: Grilled chicken or salmon with vegetable of your choice

Moderate: Vegetable soup made with Organic vegetable, chicken or beef broth with your choice of vegetables...grated carrots, green beans, celery, onions, mushrooms, whatever you have in the house. Add quinoa, rice pasta or beans. Have baked sweet potato on the side or sardines on crackers.

Weekend Impress Company or family recipe: Pistachio and broccoli pesto crusted salmon

- cup of pistachio,
- 1 garlic clove
- 2/3 cup of broccoli steam trimmed
- 1 cup of basil leaves
- 2 tbs olive oil
- 1 tbsp pine nuts
- 3 - 4 oz wild salmon

Preheat oven to 375

Line a baking sheet with parchment paper and set aside.

Place pistachios in a blender or food processor and pulse until roughly chopped.

Transfer to bowl and set aside.

Add garlic, olive oil, pine nuts and 1 tbsp of water to food processor or blender and pulse until it is a chunky puree, add more water if needed.

Put salmon filets on prepared sheets, skin side down.

Use a spatula to evenly distribute the pesto over the filets and top each with a quarter of the pistachios.

Bake for 12 to 15 minutes or till done.

Serve with gluten free or whole grain pasta, quinoa, brown rice and/or steamed vegetable of our choice.

"To get rich never risk your health.
For it is the truth that health
is the wealth of wealth."

— Richard Baker

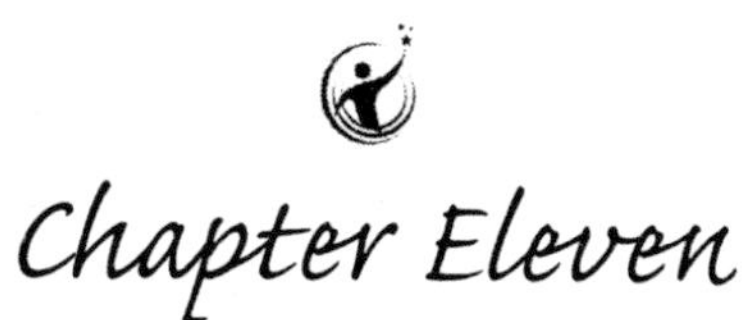

RESOURCES & LINKS FOR FURTHER RESEARCH

In addition to listing links and websites throughout this book, we are listing our favorite resources right here. The following books, videos, movies, and websites will give you quite an education. Once you start exploring, we're sure you'll find some of your own. Be forewarned that there is some controversy in theories, even among like-minded health conscious individuals. Take in all the information you can – then use your gut – "your second brain" to sort out what is best for you.

Books

- *The China Study* by T. Colin Campbell PHD
- *Earthing: The Most Important Health Discovery Ever* by Ober, Sinatra & Zucker
- *Living on High Speed* by Scott Black
- *Food Inc. (the book) How Industrial Food is Making Us Sicker, Fatter, and Poorer and What You Can do About it*, by Karl Weber
- Renee Caisse, Harry Hoxey, Mac Gerson and More
- *Health at Gunpoint* by James J. Gormley
- *Eating for Beauty* by David Wolfe. www.eatingforbeauty.com
- *What's Your Poo Telling You?* by Josh Richman and Anish Sheth
- *What's My Pee Telling Me?* by Josh Richman and Anish Sheth
- *The Gluten-Free Bible* by Jax Peters Lowell
- *Healing with Whole Foods* by Paul Pitchford
- *Seeds of Deception* by Jeffrey smith
- *The Liver Cleansing Diet* by Sandra Cabot, M.D.
- *The Detox Diet* by Elson M. Haas, M.D.

- *Discovering Raw Alkaline Cuisine* by Salomon Montezinos & Judith Castille
- *My Journey to Wellness* by Ursula Kaiser www.ursulakaiser.com
- *Raw Truth* by Jordan Rubin
- *Green Scene Diet* by Linda Berson www.greenscenediet.com
- *Raw Food Real World* by matthew Kenney & Sarma Melngailis
- *The Four Agreements* by Don Miguel Ruiz
- *Siddartha* by Herman Hesse
- *The Grain Brain* by Dr. Perlmutter
- *Against the Grain* by Jax Peters Lowell
- *Eat to Live* by Joel Fuhrman
- *The Morning Miracle* by Hal Elrod
- *The Detox Miracle Sourcebook* by Robert Morse, N.D.
- *Fats that Heal, Fats that Kill* by Udo Erasmus
- *Peace under all Circumstances* by Matthew Brownstein
- *The Virgin Diet* by JJ Virgin

Movies

- Fork Over Knives
- Food Matters
- Genetic Roulette, the Gamble of Our Lives by Jeffrey Smith
- Living Matrix: The new science of healing
- Food, Inc., the documentary.
- Cancer the Forbidden Cures A film by Massimo Mazzucco
- The GMO Trilogy by Jeffrey Smith

YouTube

- Cancer Cure Hemp Oil by Rick Simpson https://www.youtube.com/watch?v=_nm7nqUigFA
- Dr. William Li on you tube - great presentation:
- Can we eat to starve cancer A talk on food synergy and antiangiogenesis
- Energy Routine by Donna Eden: http://www.youtube.com/watch?v=Vr-FEoY440g

The two links below are helpful with the healing process, stress reduction and aligning the body.

- Tapping the Healer within– Roger Callahan www.TFTtramaRelief.wordpress.com
- Donna Eden's Energy Healing Routine http://www.youtube.com/watch?v=gffKhttrRw

Websites

- Donna Eden: www.innersource.net
- Jon Barron Report: http://www.jonbarron.org/article/energy-life
- Dr. Joseph Mercola: www.mercola.com/articles
- Sayer Ji: www.greenmedinfo.com
- Brad's Raw Chips: www.bradsrawchips.com (Gluten free vegan chips)
- www.ursulakaiser.com
- Mas Mat: www.holistichealthpemf.com
- www.undergroundhealth.com
- www.marchagainstmonsanto.com
- www.drfurhman.com
- www.mindvalley.com
- http://www.resilientcommunities.com/fermentation-is-the-new-canning/
- www.mypurium.com/healthandbeauty For a GMO-free, soy-free, synthetic-free, dairy-free cleanse! (use code healthandbeauty for a $50.00 coupon)

We've taken the liberty to include a link here to a website outlining a drink called Liquid Biocell that acts exactly as Dr. William Li explains in his Youtube presentation. The combination of the ingredients of Liquid Biocell make it 10x more effective than taking the ingredients one by one.

- www.liquidbiocell.com/carlene